W9-BXX-685

Anxiety-Free Kids

An Interactive Guide for Parents and Children

BONNIE ZUCKER, PSY.D.

Illustrated by David Parker

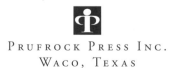

PRUFROCK PRESS INC.
WACO, TEXAS

Library of Congress Cataloging-in-Publication Data

Zucker, Bonnie, 1974-
  Anxiety-free kids : an interactive guide for parents and children / by Bonnie Zucker.
      p. cm.
  Includes bibliographical references.
  ISBN-13: 978-1-59363-343-1 (pbk.)
  ISBN-10: 1-59363-343-2 (pbk.)
  1. Anxiety in children. 2. Cognitive therapy for children. I. Title.
  RJ506.A58Z83 2009
  616.85'223--dc22

                          2008034082

Copyright © 2009, Bonnie Zucker, Psy.D., All Rights Reserved
Edited by Lacy Compton
Illustrated by David Parker
Cover and Layout Design by Marjorie Parker

ISBN-13: 978-1-59363-343-1
ISBN-10: 1-59363-343-2

No part of this book may be reproduced, translated, stored in a retrieval system, or transmitted, in any form or by any means, electronic, mechanical, photocopying, microfilming, recording, or otherwise, without written permission from the publisher.

Printed in the United States of America.

At the time of this book's publication, all facts and figures cited are the most current available. All telephone numbers, addresses, and Web site URLs are accurate and active. All publications, organizations, Web sites, and other resources exist as described in the book, and all have been verified. The author and Prufrock Press Inc. make no warranty or guarantee concerning the information and materials given out by organizations or content found at Web sites, and we are not responsible for any changes that occur after this book's publication. If you find an error, please contact Prufrock Press Inc.

Prufrock Press Inc.
P.O. Box 8813
Waco, TX 76714-8813
Phone: (800) 998-2208
Fax: (800) 240-0333
http://www.prufrock.com

I dedicate this to my husband Brian, who truly is my everything. Sharing this journey with you brings me the utmost joy and the greatest of all gifts.

And to my Mother, who taught me my two greatest lessons: how to love and how to be compassionate.

Contents

Acknowledgements

WRITING this book has been an incredibly rewarding experience. This is in large part due to the unending support I have received from my clients, colleagues, family, and friends throughout the entire process.

More than 10 years ago, I discovered my love for the treatment of anxiety disorders. Since that time, I have had the privilege of helping many children and adults who entrusted me with their well-being. This is a privilege for which I am eternally grateful. They have taught me so much about life from their ability to grow and achieve psychological freedom. Their resilience and strength are beyond impressive. Their progress is at the root of my motivation to write this book.

One of the most valuable aspects of being in this wonderful field of psychology is the ability to share it with such outstanding colleagues. I have had the good fortune to receive a great deal of consistent support and encouragement from them. My colleagues have shown confidence in me and many have allowed me to become a stronger clinician. Dr. Bernard Vittone and Dr. Mary Alvord are chief among them. By guiding me and believing in me, they both have contributed immensely to my success in practice and in this book. I am forever grateful that I have them in my life. A special thank you to Dr. Vittone for sharing his expertise in the medication portion of the parent book. Thank you to the Alvord/Baker staff for their enthusiasm during each exciting phase of this book's progress. I deeply appreciate each one of you.

I thank Drs. Rudy Bauer, Bill Lee, Bill Stixrud, and Barry Wolfe, all of whom have contributed to my growth, both personally and professionally. Your insights and perspectives have influenced me greatly. A special thank you to Dr. John McPherrin, who taught me how to be authentic and real with clients. I cannot thank Rich Weinfeld enough for connecting me with Prufrock, for demonstrating such confidence in me, and for his kindness and enthusiasm. Finally, I want to thank Dr. Harvey Parker, who is the reason why I became a psychologist. His warmth, compassionate nature, and mastery of cognitive behavioral therapy make him an extraordinary psychologist and a phenomenal person. I am beyond grateful to have had his influence.

Thank you to Dr. Judith Rapoport and Dr. Golda Ginsburg for their willingness to review and support this book. Their dedication to childhood anxiety disorders and expertise in the field is exceptional. I am honored to have had them as reviewers.

Lacy Compton, my editor at Prufrock, has been a pleasure to work with from the beginning. Her enthusiasm for this project and her superb skill as an editor resulted in major improvements to the book. I am extremely grateful for her contributions and guidance.

My family and friends have been so incredible and have provided endless encouragement through each phase of this book's development. My husband, Brian, has shared my passion for this project and has supported me at every level. He has demonstrated unconditional belief in me and my work as a psychologist, and has been patient and understanding during the many evenings and Sundays I have worked on this book (though admittedly it was to his advantage during football season!). Most of all, he has given me a foundation of love, respect, and best friendship from which all of my success grows and for which I am eternally grateful.

My mother has been a constant source of love and encouragement throughout my life. The direction she has provided, the confidence and security she has given, and the model of strength and goodness she has demonstrated have been instrumental in helping me to carve my own path in life and to become the person I am today. She has always cheered me on and taught me how to be resilient.

Thank you to Ilene and Norm who have celebrated my achievements and have provided me with unconditional love and support. I will forever be grateful for the sisterhood and best friendship that I have shared with Emily. Her enthusiasm and unfailing support mean more to me than she could ever fully realize. Lisa has provided immense encouragement, has strongly believed in this book's concept from the start, and has even been its protector at times. Thank you to Sherry, Shawn, and Scott for their unconditional love and for being so supportive. Thank you to Jessica, Denise, Amy, and Scott G. for their dear friendship and for always being so genuinely excited for me.

Finally, I am influenced every day by the light and warmth of several individuals whose love constantly surrounds me though they are no longer here. My father's memory brings me strength. The way he lived his life motivates me to succeed and work hard, and to be unwaveringly ethical. My stepfather, Irv, taught me how to live in awareness. His capacity for equality consciousness has influenced me in immeasurable ways. Most of all, his generosity of spirit and unconditional love have impacted me greatly. My grandparents, Ruth and Ben, nurtured me and nourished me with love and sweetness, and modeled how to live a good and honorable life.

Welcome to *Anxiety-Free Kids*

WELCOME to *Anxiety-Free Kids: An Interactive Guide for Parents and Children*. This book features a unique companion-book approach, offering both an information book for parents and a **tear-out** workbook for kids. Congratulations on the selection of this book's program to help your child overcome his or her anxieties, fears, and worrying behavior. It is a sign of resourcefulness and good parenting to take this step to assist your child in improving his or her experience in life, including his or her self-confidence and overall feeling of safety. This program is based on the cognitive-behavioral therapy (CBT) approach to treating anxiety disorders and it involves teaching strategies and techniques to overcome anxiety. CBT is problem-focused and solution-oriented and considers anxiety to have three components: physiological reactions, faulty and irrational thoughts, and avoidance or other nervous behaviors. It goes beyond figuring out the *causes* of the anxiety and primarily focuses on how to treat it. CBT is proactive and includes developing a detailed plan for overcoming the three parts of anxiety.

The need for a companion-book approach, including a book for the child and a parallel book for his or her parent(s), is based on the belief that the most comprehensive approach to treating a child's problem involves integrating the system in which the child lives. The field of psychology calls this a *family systems approach*, and research shows that it is a very effective way of treating the child's problem. By this, I mean that your child can use your help, but your child will do the bulk of the work while you will offer guidance, direction, encouragement, and most importantly, continuous support and praise. In addition, your insights into your child's thoughts and behaviors will be invaluable in helping him or her complete the necessary steps to overcoming anxiety and feeling better. Although other books may have a "companion" book for the child, no other series to date is designed to be read simultaneously by parent and child. The chapters in each book are paired together and address the same topic; thus, they parallel each other and are to be read separately, but together. The tear-out companion guide for kids begins immediately after your parent book begins. Simply remove the perforated pages from this book and staple each chapter together for your child. It is recommended that you and your child read and discuss one chapter at a time, and that each chapter is fully understood by your child before moving on to the next one. Also, the chapters should be read in order, without skipping any chapters.

Some children also have therapists (psychologists, psychiatrists, social workers, or professional counselors) or may begin seeing a therapist at some point. This program is intended to be all you need to help your child overcome anxiety; however, some parents will find that their child requires more than this program. If professional help is sought, this program will be an excellent supplement to your child's work with a therapist, and will guide the therapist on how to treat the anxiety from a CBT perspective. For this reason I have included the section after the Introduction entitled "A Note for Your Therapist."

All of the chapters include exercises at the end for you and your child to complete together. Some of these exercises include discussion topics and questions, while others include projects or activities. These exercises are essential in order to get the most out of the program. Generally, it is recommended that you and your child schedule time together once a week to discuss what you have read and to work on the activities. I encourage you to make these meetings as enjoyable as possible for your child (e.g., they can be outdoors in a park, at a favorite restaurant, or followed by a movie). Many children find such one-on-one time with parents quite valuable. If your child sees a therapist, your child should do the exercises with the therapist; you should receive feedback from the therapist about the exercises at each therapy session and review the exercises with your child after the session.

Although the word *parent* is used throughout each book, two parents or caregivers can read the chapters and the child can work with as many adults as desired on the activities/discussion exercises. This book is designed to be read by caretakers—and this includes stepparents, grandparents, foster parents, aunts, uncles, and so forth—however, for simplicity, I will refer to the reader as "parent," because this represents the most common situation. Finally, I will switch between male and female pronouns for the purpose of easy reading.

Best of luck,

Dr. Bonnie Zucker

Introduction

How to Use This Book

BEFORE we get started, let me tell you a little about how this program works. You and your child will read your respective books at the same time. The pages of the "For Kids Only Companion Guide" are perforated and easy to tear out. It is best to pull out and staple or clip together each chapter individually, and then present the chapters to your child one at a time to help him or her manage the task of reading the book. The chapters are matched up with one another and the content generally is the same, covering the same topics and issues. For example, Chapter 1 in both books is an introduction to anxiety. Your chapters typically will be longer and include additional information on how you can best assist your child through this program.

At the end of each chapter, there is an exercise designed to be completed together by you and your child. The exercises are explained in both books, but your book also contains recommendations on how to complete the exercises and get the most out of them, including how to make it a fun experience for you and your child. The exercises are an integral part of the program and are essential to its success. Appendix A provides an overview of the program in table form and this allows you and your child to check off when each chapter and exercise has been completed.

Your child's book explains that words like *parents*, *mom*, and *dad* are used interchangeably to describe who is completing this program with him or her, yet clarifies that other caring adults can use it too.

Finally, although I would like to think that children will be excited to read this book and be motivated solely by the prospect of feeling better, sometimes a little prompting is necessary. This may involve rewarding your child for each chapter he or she reads or for each exercise the two of you complete. I do not encourage paying your child for reading this book. However, I see nothing wrong with rewarding him or her with a privilege, such as computer time or play time or allowing him or her to choose a small prize from a "reward treasure chest" (get a box, make a personalized label for it, such as "Brian's Box of Bonuses," and fill it with small toys from the dollar store, bubble gum, homemade coupons for renting a movie of his or her choice, and so forth). In the end, the most important thing is that the child reads the chapters and completes the exercises. As always, verbal praise is of utmost importance, and once we get to the exposure phase, your child is going to need a great deal of it.

OK, let's get started!

Don't forget!
1. Tear out the "For Kids Only Companion Guide" and staple or clip each chapter together.
2. Give your child one chapter at a time. Read your respective chapters at the same time.
3. Complete the exercise at the end of each chapter together.
4. Use rewards if necessary.

A Note for Your Child's Therapist

WELCOME to *Anxiety-Free Kids*! This two-book, companion approach offers an excellent guide for you, your child client, and the child's family. I designed this book to be used either as a self-help book or as a supplement to the child's therapy. Using a cognitive-behavioral therapy (CBT) framework, the child and his parent are directed through the various steps to overcoming the child's anxiety. Six anxiety disorders are addressed: generalized anxiety disorder, separation anxiety disorder, social phobia, specific phobia, obsessive-compulsive disorder, and panic disorder. The CBT can be integrated into whatever other work you are doing, or orientation you are taking, with the child.

The child and parent read eight chapters together and then the parent's section includes two additional chapters. Each chapter includes an exercise at the end. It is my recommendation that you complete the exercises with the child during your session time (e.g., make self-talk note cards with him or her in session). You may or may not choose to include parents in the process of completing the exercises; at minimum, parents should be asked to contribute examples of the child's anxious and avoidance behaviors and should receive feedback on the exercises and what was accomplished in the session. I also highly recommend that you help the child learn the thinking errors and identify which ones she uses most often when she is anxious.

Best of luck,

Dr. Bonnie Zucker

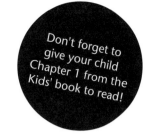

Don't forget to give your child Chapter 1 from the Kids' book to read!

CHAPTER

1

Anxiety

What It Is and What to Do About It

Ten-year-old Kimberly worries a lot. She worries about her homework, her dog, her house, and what other kids think about her. Kimberly has a hard time adjusting to unexpected changes. Last week when her Mom picked her up from school and told her about her dentist appointment, Kimberly had a meltdown and became very upset because Mom didn't tell her about it the day before. The appointment had to be rescheduled. When doing homework Kimberly often gets very nervous about not having enough time to finish it, even though it usually takes about an hour, and sometimes becomes so stressed that she cannot concentrate or organize her thoughts. She worries that someone will break into her house and possibly kidnap her, and each time she approaches her house, her heart starts to beat fast. For this reason, Kimberly refuses to be the first person to walk into the house and has her Mom or Dad go in first and check that no one has broken in. Kimberly also checks on her dog many times each day to make sure he is OK and didn't run out of the house. Kimberly gets a lot of stomachaches and headaches from all of her worrying.

KIMBERLY, and many children like her, suffers from an anxiety disorder. Her childhood is filled with worries and feelings of uneasiness. Kimberly's parents struggle to make her feel calm and comfortable, and feel at a loss of what to do to help her. If your child has anxiety like Kimberly, or has a different type of anxiety, then this book is for you. You and your child will receive guidance on how to become aware of what his anxiety symptoms are and how they can be addressed and overcome in a step-by-step fashion.

In this chapter, your child will learn the following:

1. common symptoms of anxiety,
2. how to differentiate normal versus problematic anxiety,
3. the three parts of anxiety, and
4. how to address each of the three parts of anxiety.

These topics will be addressed in this chapter, and the exercise that you will complete with your child after you each read Chapter 1 of your respective books will be reviewed. This chapter also will include descriptions of the different anxiety disorders, an explanation of the cognitive-behavioral therapy (CBT) approach to treating anxiety disorders, how best to use this program with your child and what to say to him or her when implementing it, and advice on determining if your child requires professional help and/ or medication.

Anxiety: Its Symptoms and Disorders

Anxiety is the experience of feeling nervous, worried, scared, or afraid, and it is the opposite of feeling relaxed. All children and adults feel anxious at times. Sometimes anxiety arises as a result of an event, such as when you are driving and almost hit the car in front of you. Sometimes it appears out of the blue. Our capacity for anxiety is a survival mechanism that allows us to react quickly in a threatening situation by providing a physical reaction known as the "flight or fight" response. In addition, anxiety can be a motivator and can help us get things done in a timely manner. For example,

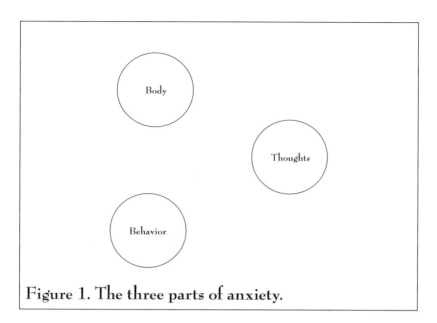

Figure 1. The three parts of anxiety.

the anxiety associated with having to pass a test serves as a motivator for studying for it.

Anxiety involves three parts: physiological feelings (body), thoughts, and behavior. Typically, the behavior associated with anxiety is avoidance. When children and adults avoid anxiety-provoking situations, such avoidance breeds self-doubt. Over time, the repetitive practice of self-doubting impacts and even damages one's self-esteem.

The diagram in Figure 1 is included in your child's chapter to help him or her conceptualize the three parts of anxiety.

In order to understand and treat anxiety, we need to understand and address the three parts. Each part will be discussed in greater detail in later chapters. Common physical (*body*) symptoms of anxiety are:

- ▶ rapid heart rate,
- ▶ shallow breathing,
- ▶ muscle tension,
- ▶ sweating,

- difficulty swallowing,
- choking sensations,
- dizziness,
- stomachaches,
- shaking, and
- feeling detached from one's body or from reality.

Somatic complaints are physical symptoms that are psychological in nature (have no organic or medical cause) and include stomachaches, headaches, and general aches and pains. If your child displays what appear to be somatic complaints, I recommend that he or she receives a comprehensive physical exam to rule out any underlying physical problem even though you may feel the cause is psychological.

The cognitive (or *thoughts*) part of anxiety includes the following: worries, thinking errors, negative self-talk, and a perceived irrational threat. Anxious children often will use "what if's" when they worry about bad things happening to them or to their parents or loved ones. Worries also may center on performance in social situations, such as test anxiety and social anxiety. Examples of thinking errors, also known as cognitive distortions, include:

- "Other kids will laugh at me if I raise my hand and give the wrong answer,"
- "I should get all A's in school. Getting a B means that I am a failure," and
- "It happened to her so it will happen to me."

As mentioned above, the *behavior* part of anxiety typically includes avoidance behavior. However, if the child does not avoid the anxiety-provoking situation, he or she will endure it with extreme distress. Examples of avoidance include:

- not going near the feared object (dogs, injections);
- refusing to separate from mom or dad;
- not sleeping alone;

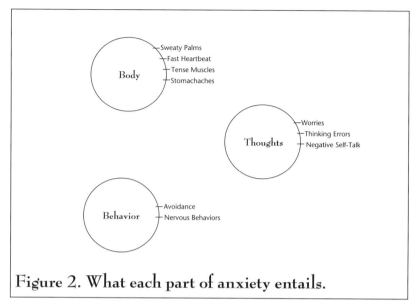

Figure 2. What each part of anxiety entails.

- ▶ refusing to go over to a friend's house for a sleepover; and
- ▶ refusing to go to school.

Children with anxiety often display nervous behaviors, such as seeking reassurance (asking a parent or caregiver to tell them that they will be OK), checking behaviors (e.g., checking that doors are locked, checking that parents are OK), picking/pulling behaviors, crying, freezing up, and having a meltdown or tantrum.

Now let's look at the three parts again, taking into account what each entails. (See Figure 2.)

Anxiety goes from being "normal" to being a problem or disorder in need of treatment when it causes a significant interference in the child's life. This is the key factor in determining if your child needs help in dealing with her anxiety. If the anxiety interferes with your child's academic or social performance (e.g., it prevents your child from going to school, birthday parties, or sleepovers, or from sleeping alone at night, or if it renders her unable to concentrate at school due to focus on worries), or interferes with your child's ability to enjoy life (e.g., daily stomachaches or headaches, persistent worry, negative self-image), this is a good indication that her anxiety has become a disorder. A fear of something becomes a phobia when it involves avoidance of the feared object or situation *or* if exposure to the feared object or situation is endured with extreme distress, and causes a significant impairment in her life.

Anxiety Disorders

Anxiety disorders are the most common form of psychological disorders in children and adults. An estimated 6–17% of children, or about 1 in 10, suffer from an anxiety disorder (Costello & Angold, 1995). Approximately 20% of children and adolescents will meet the criteria for an anxiety disorder at some point in their lives (Shaffer et al., 1996). Research has demonstrated that an untreated anxiety disorder in childhood often persists into adulthood. Anxiety is considered to be an internalizing disorder, meaning that its symptoms are not always evident from the perspective of an outsider. This is in contrast with externalizing disorders, such as disruptive or aggressive behaviors, which are hard to miss. It also is important to note that anxiety disorders (specifically generalized anxiety disorder) and Attention Deficit/Hyperactivity Disorder (ADHD) have symptoms that overlap. For example, restlessness, difficulty concentrating, difficulty sustaining focus, and one's mind going blank are all symptoms of both disorders. Consider the difficulty associated with trying to balance your checkbook while fearing that at any moment, someone will break into your house and harm you. Thus, making a differential diagnosis is very important, as the treatments are different. In particular, the medication treatment typically used for ADHD (stimulant medication such as Ritalin and Adderall) may impair the treatment of anxiety disorders, as these medications can result in an increase in anxiety symptoms.

There are several different anxiety disorders listed in the *Diagnostic and Statistical Manual of Mental Disorders*, fourth edition (*DSM-IV*; the Bible of psychiatric disorders). When an individual meets the criteria for one disorder and for another disorder, this is called *comorbidity*. The most common comorbid disorder for an anxiety disorder is another anxiety disorder. Research shows that, on average, between 50–80% of children and adolescents with an anxiety disorder also meet the criteria for one or more additional anxiety disorders (Curry, March, & Hervey, 2004). Children and adolescents with anxiety disorders have a 17–50% chance of also having a comorbid, or co-occurring, diagnosis of a depressive disorder (Curry et al., 2004). In addition, children with other diagnoses can have a comorbid anxiety disorder; for example, a National Institute of Mental Health (NIMH) study found that about 35% of children with Attention Deficit/Hyperactivity Disorder (ADHD) have an anxiety disorder (Jensen et al., 2001).

The six disorders that I most often see in children include:

▸ Generalized Anxiety Disorder (GAD),
▸ Separation Anxiety Disorder (SAD),
▸ Social Phobia (SoP),
▸ Specific Phobia (SP),
▸ Obsessive-Compulsive Disorder (OCD), and
▸ Panic Disorder (PD).

Each disorder is discussed in greater detail in Chapter 10, but a brief overview of the disorders below should help you as you work with your child in this book. Remember that it also may be beneficial to read more about the disorder you suspect your child may have by turning to Chapter 10 before beginning the program.

Generalized anxiety disorder (GAD) is characterized by excessive worry that occurs more days than not for at least 6 months and is difficult to contain. The symptoms include restlessness, being easily fatigued, difficulty concentrating, irritability, muscle tension, sleep disturbance, and physical complaints.

Separation anxiety disorder (SAD) involves excessive distress when the child is separated from home or from attachment figures or when separation is anticipated. The child often worries about harm befalling major attachment figures, like parents, and may refuse to go to school or elsewhere in efforts to avoid separation. Children with SAD often refuse to sleep in their own beds or without their parent(s) present, and may exhibit physical symptoms or complaints when separation occurs or is anticipated.

Social phobia (SoP) is the fear of social or performance situations in which the child will be exposed to unfamiliar people or possible scrutiny by others. A child with social phobia fears that he or she will act in a way that will be embarrassing or humiliating, and tends to believe that there is a great likelihood that a negative event or outcome will occur in social or performance situations.

Specific phobias (SP) are pretty easy to identify. This is what people generally think of when they say someone has a phobia. Specific phobias involve marked and persistent fear that is excessive or unreasonable and occurs in the presence of, anticipation of, or exposure to a specific object or situation. Exposure to the phobic situation is either avoided or endured with extreme distress. The DSM-IV lists five subtypes of specific phobias: animal type, natural environment type (storms, heights, water), blood-injection-injury type, situational type (flying, elevators, enclosed places), or other type.

Obsessive compulsive disorder (OCD) is characterized by the presence of obsessions or compulsions, but usually both occur. Obsessions are intrusive thoughts, images, or impulses. For example, contamination fears, harm to others, and symmetry urges (everything needs to be perfectly ordered and aligned) are all obsessions. Compulsions or rituals are repetitive intentional behaviors or mental acts performed in response to an obsession. For example, washing, checking, touching in a certain way, counting, and ordering all are compulsions or rituals. The compulsions are performed in order to reduce the anxiety caused by obsessions. To meet the criteria for OCD, the symptoms must cause distress and must either be time-consuming (taking at least one hour a day) or cause a significant interference with the child's normal routine, academic functioning, or social interaction.

Finally, *panic disorder* (PD) includes the presence of panic attacks and a fear of having additional panic attacks. Situations in which the child is afraid of having an attack often are avoided. A panic attack is a terrifying experience in which the individual is consumed with at least four of the following symptoms (listed in the DSM-IV), most of which are experienced as physical in nature:

1. palpitations, pounding heart, or accelerated heart rate;
2. sweating;
3. trembling or shaking;
4. sensations of shortness of breath or smothering;
5. feeling of choking;
6. chest pain or discomfort;
7. nausea or abdominal distress;
8. feeling dizzy, unsteady, lightheaded, or faint;
9. de-realization (feelings of unreality) or depersonalization (being detached from oneself);
10. fear of losing control or going crazy;
11. fear of dying;
12. paresthesias (numbness or tingling sensations); or
13. chills or hot flushes.

In order to become familiar with the different anxiety disorders, try to identify which anxiety disorder is described in the six examples listed below.

▸ At the age of 6, James was in his backyard helping his father pull weeds from the garden. As he pulled out one large weed, a garden snake jumped out at him and landed on his stomach before falling to the ground. After this experience, James became afraid of snakes. He began to worry about encountering a snake. Whenever he was outdoors, he would be on guard looking for snakes. If he heard an animal moving in the bushes, he would run away, fearing that it was a snake. As years passed, James's fear grew and grew. When he watched a scene from one of the *Harry Potter* movies that had a snake in it, he became terrified. He refused to go to his friend's house because the friend kept a snake as a pet. James even avoided eating cucumbers as they reminded him of snakes! Sometimes James would even feel sick to his stomach just thinking of snakes, and wouldn't eat spaghetti or other foods that were "snake-like." He came in for therapy at the age of 12 as his symptoms were continuing to get worse.

▸ One night before bed, Emily was in her room when she suddenly felt like she was choking, and couldn't breathe. It seemed to come out of nowhere. She immediately ran to get her mother and told her mother what was happening, and that she thought she could be dying. Her heart was pounding, she felt dizzy, and began to feel a flush of hot and then cold running through her body. As this was happening, she worried about what was happening to her, and felt like it wasn't real. This feeling made her even more afraid and she began sobbing as her mother held her and rubbed her back. Eventually, Emily was able to catch her breath and calm down, though she still felt shaky for a few more hours. The next night as she was getting ready for bed, Emily told her mother that she worried it would happen again. She decided not to go to a sleepover party the next weekend because she did not want to go through this again when she was not in the comfort of her own home and with her family.

▸ Billy was a very bright 9-year-old with a phenomenal imagination. He spent his time designing very sophisticated and creative games, and was always happy when he worked on his games. Despite being so bright, Billy had a learning disability and took a very long time to do writing assignments at school. Some of his teachers did not understand that he had a learning disability, and would punish him for not having all his work done. At times, he even had to stay in from recess to finish his work. This made Billy feel very uncomfortable and embarrassed. He began to worry about getting in trouble and having to stay back. As a result, Billy would daydream and had trouble focusing on his work. He had very tense muscles, found it difficult to go to sleep, and often would stay up most of the night worrying. Billy complained to his mother and father about headaches and feeling tired. His worry interfered with his ability to concentrate and focus on his schoolwork. Sometimes he would be so worried that he would not want to go to school.

▸ Carlos was a responsible, bright, and athletic 12-year-old with lots of friends. His parents described him as shy and quiet, but well-liked by others. Carlos reported that he felt very uncomfortable at school, especially during class and basketball games. In particular, he worried that he would speak in class and say something "stupid," and that others would laugh at him. He worried so much that he never raised his hand and dreaded the times that a teacher called on him. Carlos also worried that he would forget about a test or quiz and that he would fail and the teacher would get mad at him. When playing basketball, he was terrified that he would make a mistake and embarrass himself. As a result, he often missed basketball games.

▸ Ten-year-old Ruth spent a lot of time worrying that she would get sick. Specifically, she thought that she would get sick by getting germs from others. When at a sleepover, Ruth refused to eat chips out of a bowl that others had touched. She never ate anything homemade, especially baked goods, or anything from the school cafeteria. Using public bathrooms was so uncomfortable for her, that she often "held it" until she got home. When she did use public bathrooms, she did her best not to touch anything there—she used her foot to flush the toilet and used paper towels or her sleeve to touch the faucet and door handles. If Ruth accidentally touched anything in the bathroom, even the walls of the stall, she would insist that her mother wash her clothes immediately once they got home. She wanted her mom to wash everything twice, to make sure the germs were gone. Even though she didn't really know why she was so afraid of germs, sometimes she would become so distressed about getting germs on her, that she would stay at home in her room all day.

▶   Thelma became very anxious when she would separate from her mother. It even bothered her if her mother went out to the front of the house to take out the trash. In public places, Thelma refused to go to the bathroom alone, and insisted that someone went with her. At home, she always left the bathroom door wide open. She worried that something bad would happen to her or to her mother. When her mother left the room, she would sing to Thelma so Thelma would know which room her mother was in at all times. If her mother would go out to art class, Thelma would get very sick and many times, she would vomit. Her mother felt so bad about this that she decided to bring Thelma with her to art class.

Answers: James meets the criteria for a Specific Phobia; Emily has Panic Disorder; Billy has Generalized Anxiety Disorder; Carlos has Social Phobia; Ruth has Obsessive-Compulsive Disorder; and Thelma has Separation Anxiety Disorder.

What to Do About It: Cognitive-Behavioral Therapy

Cognitive-behavioral therapy (CBT) is the most empirically supported approach in the treatment of anxiety disorders in children and adults. This means that the research on the different types of therapies used to treat anxiety disorders has shown that the cognitive-behavioral approach is the most effective. In all honesty, I love it. We all have our passions, and you may think it is a little odd that mine is CBT, but it really is *that* good! It is problem-focused and solution-oriented, practical, short-term (e.g., an average of 12–16 sessions), oriented with providing the client with useful coping strategies and techniques, and it helps children change their thinking patterns that not only help them with their anxiety now, but theoretically can serve to prevent problems from developing in the future (many anxieties develop out of thinking errors and irrational thinking). In addition, by challenging one's thinking patterns, CBT can result in a significant improvement in one's self-esteem and self-confidence (e.g., by teaching common thinking errors and replacement thoughts).

Although other therapies can be helpful, research consistently finds that CBT is the best approach to effectively treating anxiety in children and adults (Christophersen & Mortweet, 2001; Hollon, Stewart, & Strunk, 2006). I believe this is largely due to CBT's focus on solving problems and providing strategies and techniques for doing so. Other approaches, such as classic psychoanalytic therapy, are less structured, less directive, and often do not involve the teaching of strategies or techniques. Rather, the psychoanalytic approach is aimed at understanding the causes of the anxiety disorder, including the unconscious experience of the child. In my view, this is unhelpful for a child with anxiety who needs direction and techniques to cope with his symptoms.

So, what is CBT anyway? Well, you already have been introduced to the cognitive-behavioral understanding that anxiety involves three parts: cognitions, behaviors, and feelings. Other books may call the feelings a physical or physiological component—but it's all the same. CBT considers that thoughts and feelings/moods are related, and that you can change the way you feel by changing the way you think. This point is very important to remember when helping your child with his or her anxiety: If we can change the way we *think*, we can change the way we *feel*. So, if we think differently, we can reduce our feelings of anxiety. Of course, we also have to work on the behaviors associated with anxiety, such as avoidance, to treat the disorder comprehensively. In terms of thinking patterns, CBT theorizes that individuals with anxiety make thinking errors (I refer to them as *thinking mistakes* in your child's book) and that these errors cause, maintain, and strengthen the anxiety. CBT teaches the child to replace these thinking errors with rational responses (reality-based, logical thoughts), a practice particularly helpful in addressing worries and phobias. Changing the way you think also involves altering one's inner dialogue or *self-talk*: changing negative thoughts to coping thoughts. CBT helps decrease anxiety through practicing relaxation and calm breathing. Finally, the behavioral part of CBT explains that one's anxiety is maintained and strengthened by avoidance behaviors. To treat this, the child needs to be *systematically desensitized* (or gradually exposed) to the anxiety-provoking situations, starting with the ones that elicit the least anxiety and gradually moving up toward the ones that seem most frightening. This is consistent with the "face your fears" mentality. When the child is exposed to the anxiety-provoking situation, he or she will experience anxiety. However, if the child stays in the situation, the anxiety will begin to decrease. This process is called *habituation*. For example, if a child with a dog phobia spends one hour a day with different dogs, this child will get used to being with dogs and no longer will feel anxious around them. Then the child will begin to relax when he or she is around dogs, pairing together dogs and a relaxed feeling.

Sounds pretty good, right? Well, the best part is that the program in this book is based on cognitive-behavioral theory and therapy. The techniques your child will learn to use to cope with anxiety and the exercises you will complete together all are rooted in CBT.

In order to effectively treat anxiety, all three parts must be addressed. Prior to considering each part, we need to talk about the importance of externalizing the anxiety. As discussed earlier, anxiety is an internalizing disorder, and children feel like the anxiety is a part of them. The goal is for this to shift so the child can view anxiety as something separate from him or her. One way to do this is to encourage your child to identify his or her worries and nervous feelings as anxiety. For instance, when you hear your child expressing separation worries, say to him: "That's the anxiety talking. When you feel worried about something bad happening to Mommy, it's the anxiety talking to you." In Chapter 4, you and your child will work together to make a list called, "When My Anxiety Talks, It Says . . . " The more you emphasize this, the easier it will be for your child to identify the symptoms of anxiety and to work toward overcoming them. Your child will learn that it's her against the anxiety or fear, and that each time she listens to the fear and avoids a situation, the fear wins and becomes stronger. One key component is helping your child understand that to beat the anxiety and win, he or she will need to learn that anxiety itself it not that scary. Although anxiety is uncomfortable, it is not dangerous. This logic is important to grasp and seems a bit counterintuitive. Because anxiety is unpleasant, we try to avoid it; however, in avoiding it, we become more anxious. You and your child will come to see that, in breaking the anxiety cycle, he will have to be able to tolerate some anxious experiences (e.g., when facing his fears). Helping your child to understand the symptoms of his anxiety disorder and the principle of learning not to fear the anxiety will lay the foundation for facing his fears.

We will go through the three parts of anxiety (body, thoughts, and behavior) in order, starting with the body. You and your child will learn deep breathing, progressive muscle relaxation (PMR), and guided imagery relaxation. For the thoughts component, your child will learn positive self-talk, how to identify and replace thinking errors, and how to conquer (or master) worry. She will learn the difference between realistic and unrealistic thinking, and that her fears are irrational. We also will discuss self-esteem and self-confidence, which will improve once your child begins to successfully face her fears. For the behavior part, you and your child will learn the Face Your Fears approach, which states that one must face his or her fears to overcome them. Thus, your child will learn that avoidance of anxiety-provoking situations is not the answer to dealing with

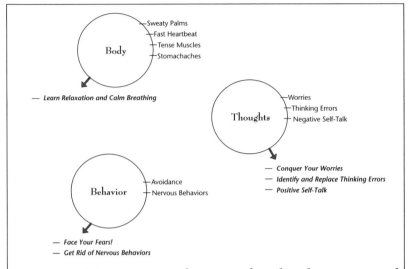

Figure 3. Treatment techniques for the three parts of anxiety.

fears. We also will work on understanding and eliminating nervous behaviors, such as reassurance seeking.

Figure 3 is an extension of Figure 2, with the treatment techniques for each part noted.

It is essential that parents are empathic and understanding during this process of treating the anxiety disorder. It is critical that parents do not blame, criticize, or tease their child for their anxiety disorder in any way, and that siblings are prevented from doing the same. Many parents interpret their child's anxiety-related behaviors as a product of oppositionality. However, this is rarely the case. The majority of the time, a child's seemingly oppositional behavior is a direct expression of his anxiety. It is important to conceptualize these behaviors as part of the anxiety disorder. For example, avoidance behaviors, resistance to change, and inflexibility all are common behaviors associated with a childhood anxiety disorder.

Finally, let me provide some guidance on how to make this book work best for you and your child. First of all, providing support, encouragement, and communicating confidence in your child and in his ability to face his fears is one of the greatest gifts you could give to your anxious child in his life. As his parent, your child looks to you for signals and cues that he can charter into new territory and not be harmed. It is up to you to confirm this for him and emphasize that, not only will he not be harmed, but he will be helped and strengthened by taking what will feel like a huge risk. Of the children with anxiety disorders, those whose parents demonstrate that they fully believe in their child and his ability to master the anxiety do the best in therapy and have the best outcomes. I also recommend using humor with your child, staying positive, and reminding your child to use the strategies and tools he learns from reading his book. Finally, I encourage you to talk to your child about the process that is involved in overcoming his anxieties. For example, making the following comments will help:

▶ (When doing relaxation): "You are practicing your calm breathing because you are going to use it when you begin to face your fears. You are doing a great job preparing yourself. I'm so proud of you!"

▶ (When doing self-talk note cards): "We are making these positive self-talk note cards to help you change the things you say to yourself when you are nervous. Using the note cards will help you feel better and calm."

▶ (When making hierarchy): "Together, we are making a list of all the things that are hard to do because they make you feel nervous or scared. We are doing this because eventually you will face these fears, one step at a time. Remember that the book explains that you never will be forced to do these things. But I *will* encourage you to do them."

▶ (When facing their fears): "I know this is so hard for you, and that you feel nervous. But, remember what the book (or Dr. Zucker) says about this: You are not expected to like the nervous feeling, but you can handle it, it is not harmful to you. And, it will go away and it will get easier with practice.

I am so proud of you and you should be very, very proud of yourself."

▸ (When refusing to provide reassurance, which may be one of the steps on their hierarchy): "I know this is hard for you, but we both know that I can't _____ (e.g., give you the answer you want to hear, tell you it will be OK, tell you what we're doing tomorrow, let you sleep in my bed, tell you who is going to be there). If I do _____ (same as first blank), it will make you feel better right now, but will make the overall anxiety much, much worse. Remember, you have to go through being nervous before it gets better. I know you can do it."

It is always appropriate to answer your child's questions about the process and the purpose behind doing the activities that help her face her fears. However, if your child asks these questions repetitively, then it may be a symptom of anxiety (especially if asking a lot of questions is one of her reassurance-seeking behaviors). It will be important not to answer the questions over and over again. Instead, you can refer your child to her book to find the solutions.

Managing your own reaction to your child's anxiety and anxious behaviors is an important component of the treatment. Your child needs a strong foundation to help contain himself and his fears, and he will benefit from stability and a predictable reaction from you as he addresses his anxiety. Consistency in reading the chapters and doing the exercises is very important, particularly for anxious children who are comforted by predictability. Many parents have told me that they use the strategies their child learns for their own benefit, and many practice relaxation and use calm breathing to manage their own anxiety. Because anxiety disorder tends to run in families, you may find that either you or someone else in your child's family also suffers from an anxiety disorder. If this is the case, it may be equally important to get your own treatment or treatment for other family members living in the home.

What About Professional Help and Medication?

Using this self-help program is an excellent first step in addressing the anxiety, and it is my goal and hope that this will be enough—that by the time you complete it, your child no longer will suffer from an anxiety disorder, and you and your family will be free from the limitations associated with it. Of course, you may be using this book in conjunction with ongoing psychotherapy, which can be very helpful. If you are using this as a form of self-help for your child, and at the completion of the program your child continues to have symptoms that cause an interference in his or her life, I recommend that you seek professional assistance. In this case, please refer to the last pages of this book for resources, or ask your child's pediatrician or school for a recommendation.

There are two main classes of medications used to treat anxiety in children and adults: *antidepressants* (which include SSRIs, or selective serotonin reuptake inhibitors; SNRIs, or serotonin norepinephrine reuptake inhibitors; TCAs, or tricyclic antidepressants; and "atypical" antidepressants) and *antianxiety medications* (which include benzodiazepines and buspirone). Both classes have been shown to decrease symptoms of anxiety and generally are considered to be safe. Antidepressants take a longer time to take effect, usually requiring 2–6 weeks before reaching a therapeutic level, and must be taken daily. Antianxiety medications take effect immediately and, in some cases, can be taken on an "as-needed" basis. In many cases, these medications will be prescribed in combination. Sometimes, an antipsychotic medication will be added to enhance the efficiency of the antidepressants or antianxiety medications. If prescribed, it usually is a very low dose and often will be discontinued once the child's symptoms improve. Psychiatrists and pediatricians (both of whom are medical doctors) are able to prescribe these medications. Table 1 lists commonly prescribed antidepressants, antianxiety medications, and the newer antipsychotics, as well as their common side effects.

Table 1
Antianxiety Medications

Type	Brand (Generic) Name	Side Effects
Antidepressants		
SSRIs	Celexa (citalopram) Lexapro (escitalopram) Luvox (fluvoxamine) Paxil (paroxetine) Prozac (fluoxetine) Zoloft (sertraline)	Stomachaches, diarrhea, tremor, initial increased anxiety, agitation, irritability, headaches, sedation, trouble sleeping, low sex drive, erectile dysfunction
SNRIs	Cymbalta (duloxetine) Effexor (venlafaxine) Pristiq (desvenlafaxine)	Same as SSRIs
TCAs	Anafranil (clomipramine) Elavil (amitriptyline) Pamelor (nortriptyline) Tofranil (imipramine)	Dry mouth, constipation, dizziness, tremor, sedation, anxiety, weight gain
Atypicals	Desyrel (trazodone) Remeron (mirtazapine) Serzone (nefazodone) Wellbutrin (bupropion)	Drowsiness, weight gain, dry mouth, anxiety, constipation, insomnia, irritability, tremor, priapism (erection that will not go away)
Antianxiety		
Benzodiazepines	Ativan (lorazepam) Klonopin (clonazepam) Valium (diazepam) Xanax (alprazolam)	Drowsiness, fatigue, lethargy, increased anxiety, impaired coordination, memory problems, withdrawal symptoms
Other	Buspar (buspirone)	Same as Benzodiazepines
Antipsychotics	Abilify (aripiprazole) Clozaril (clozapine) Geodon (ziprasidone) Risperdal (risperidone) Seroquel (quetiapine) Zyprexa (olanzapine)	Increased appetite, weight gain, sedation, dizziness, dry mouth, blurred vision, muscle spasms, diabetes, tardive dyskinesia (repetitive, involuntary movements), restlessness, tremor

It is very important to report all side effects to your child's doctor, although many of them will subside within a few weeks of your child being on the medication. In addition to these side effects, if your child has any of the following symptoms: shortness of breath, fainting, disorientation, intense muscle tension, or fever, then contact your doctor immediately, or take your child to the emergency room.

It is good practice for a medical doctor to use a drug's side effects to the patient's advantage. For example, anxious children who have trouble sleeping or are underweight might be prescribed Remeron because it has the side effects of drowsiness and weight gain. It is important to note an SSRI's side effect of initial increased anxiety typically results from starting on a dose that is too high; in this case, lowering the dose should help. Wellbutrin should not be prescribed for individuals with eating disorders due to the risk of seizures (sometimes children with anxiety, especially OCD, can have co-occurring eating disorders). Anytime a medication is stopped, it must be done in a gradual fashion. Suddenly stopping a medication can lead to significant side effects, particularly for Effexor and Paxil, which are known for withdrawal symptoms if they are discontinued abruptly. Finally, doctors should be informed of any other health problem or condition your child may have, as this may influence which type of drug is prescribed.

The research on anxiety disorders treatment has concluded that people do just as well if they use medication *or* do CBT; however, CBT leads to better long-term results with lower incidence of relapse (Barlow, 2004; Hollon et al., 2006). Medication can lead to a greater short-term benefit, but the effects are not as strong as CBT in the long run. When making the decision to have your child begin medication, consider my two rules of thumb: (1) your child should only begin medication if, after 3 months of cognitive behavioral therapy, you, your child, and the therapist feel there has been little or no improvement and (2) your child should *only* be on medication if he or she also continues to attend therapy with a licensed therapist. I believe there is one exception to the first rule of thumb: your child may benefit from taking an immediate-acting benzodiazepine (e.g., Klonopin, Xanax) if there is an imminent situation that warrants it (e.g., your child has a fear of flying and will be flying in the very near future or your child refuses to go to school and is missing most days). If medication is used, once the child improves to the point at which the anxiety no longer meets the criteria for a disorder, and this progress is maintained for 6–12 months, he or she gradually can be taken off the medication, under the supervision of the prescribing doctor. The majority of the time, medication should not be considered a permanent treatment, but only a temporary one. Consult your doctor or a psychiatrist for more information.

In summary, anxiety disorders are the most common psychological disorder of childhood. CBT is the most effective and empirically supported treatment approach for anxiety disorders, and it views anxiety has having three components: body, thoughts, and behavior. We will address these three parts of anxiety and we will start by identifying your child's anxiety-provoking situations and avoidance behaviors in the next chapter.

Chapter 1 Exercise

Tips for Parents

1. As a reminder, exercises are to be completed by you and your child together. The exercises appear the same in your child's book, thus you'll note that the exercises in your book are written to your child.
2. When completing this exercise with your child, try to elicit as many personal examples as possible.

Fill in the Bubbles

Directions: You and your mom or dad will do this together. In each of the bubbles, write in the three parts of anxiety. Next to each part (bubble), write your own examples of your experience with anxiety. For example, you can write down what specific things happen to your body when you are anxious.

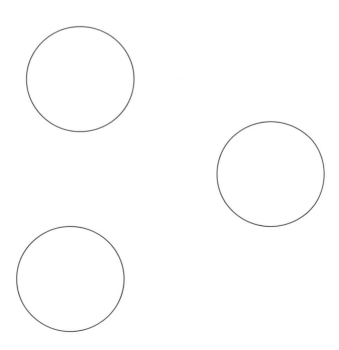

2

Making Your Team and Team Goals

Kimberly and her parents learned that she has Generalized Anxiety Disorder (GAD) and that she will need to learn how to relax her body, change the ways she thinks, and face her fears. She realized that there were a lot of things she avoided doing because they made her feel afraid or uncomfortable. Kimberly and her mom worked together to make a list of all of the situations that cause Kimberly to feel anxious or worried. They made the list into a ladder, so Kimberly could see the different steps she would take to overcome her anxiety, and note her progress along the way. Kimberly decided that her first step would be to reduce the number of times she checked on her dog to only twice a day.

I N this chapter, your child will learn the following:

1. the "Face Your Fears" philosophy,
2. a case example of Thelma who overcame her separation anxiety by facing her fears, and
3. how to form a team and make a ladder (hierarchy) for achieving goals.

These topics will be addressed in this chapter, and the exercise that you will complete with your child after you each read Chapter 2 of your respective books will be discussed. This chapter also will include a section on the importance of not providing reassurance.

This is a shorter chapter to read, but the exercise that you and your child will complete is longer than most of the other exercises in this book. The exercise (Making Your Team and Team Goals) is going to be fun and will set the stage for your child's treatment goals: facing his or her fears. It is through facing his own fears that your child will learn to overcome them and break free from the cycle of anxiety. When your child avoids situations that evoke anxiety, this is called *avoidance behavior* because she is avoiding something in reaction to the anxiety. Think about it, it makes sense. Your child's mentality is akin to:

> When I _____ (separate from Mom, raise my hand in class, go near a dog), I feel completely scared, threatened, nervous, and/or terrified, so of course I don't want to do it again.

However, each time that your child avoids something because it makes her feel anxious, *the anxiety wins* and becomes reinforced and strengthened, and *your child loses*. But each time your child does something that makes her feel anxious, *she wins* and *the anxiety loses*. It is your child against the anxiety (in the kids' companion book I call this, "You vs. Anxiety"), and it is certain that as your child faces her fears, she *will* win!

Although you learned a little about Thelma in the last chapter, the following is directly from your child's book and gives more detail about Thelma's experience, as well as her process of facing her fears:

> Eight-year-old Thelma was one of the children I worked with in therapy. She was very nice, very smart, and very

nervous about being separated from her mom. If her mom went out in the front of the house to take out the trash, Thelma would become anxious—her heart would beat fast, and she would stop doing whatever she was doing to go to the window and watch her mom. Thelma would worry that something bad would happen to her and that she wouldn't come back. Thelma also did not like to be in a different room than her mom, and when her mom would go in another room, Thelma would ask her to sing a song so Thelma would always know where she was. She refused to sleep in her own bed at night even though her mom would try to get her to sleep alone, but Thelma would cry and cry and beg her mom to be able to sleep with her. Sometimes, Thelma's mom needed to go out without her and a babysitter would come over; this upset Thelma so much that she would get sick and throw up. As soon as her mom would come home, Thelma would feel better. This made it very hard for her mom to leave the house without her!

Thelma has separation anxiety, which means that she gets very nervous and worried when she is separated from her mom and worries about bad things happening to her mom. She does her best to *avoid* being separated from her, because this is the thing that makes her feel so scared. Each time that Thelma clings onto her mother and *avoids* being separated from her, *the anxiety wins and she loses.* Even though staying near her mother helps her to feel better at the time, it actually makes the anxiety much worse overall. Thelma learned that she had to face her fears to overcome them. How did she do it?

Thelma and her team (her Mom, sister, and me, Dr. Zucker) worked together to make a list of all of the things that felt scary to her and that were hard to do. Then, Thelma and I put the list in order, from easiest to hardest, and wrote them all on a poster board, in the form of a ladder. Each step on the ladder was one of the things that was hard for her to do. Thelma learned how to relax and take deep breaths, learned that her fears were not realistic (it was perfectly safe for her mom to take out the trash), and learned what to say to herself to help herself deal with the scary thoughts and feelings. Thelma also learned that she was making thinking mistakes and worked on correcting them. Finally, she understood that she needed to face her fears, one step (or fear) at a time. She knew that when she was facing her fears, she would have to handle feeling some anxiety, but that the anxiety would go away with time and practice. Most importantly, Thelma was told that she would not have to take any of the steps until she was ready; Thelma would not be forced to face her fears. Instead, Thelma would be *encouraged* by her team to face her fear—she would be cheered on.

Thelma named her ladder "Climbing to Confidence" because she felt that her separation anxiety made her feel less confident about herself. By facing her fears, she would feel more confident. This is what Thelma's ladder looked like:

Climbing to Confidence

(top)	Mom goes out of town without you.
	Go on a sleepover at a friend's house.
	Mom goes out for the day without you.
	Go on a play date at a friend's house.
	Mom goes out for 1 hour, then 2 hours without you.
	Mom goes out for 15 minutes, then 30 minutes without you.
	Sleep in your bed alone one night this week (then 2, 4, 5, and 7 nights).
	You use a public bathroom on your own (without Mom).
	Mom takes the trash out and you stay focused on the TV.

	Mom stays upstairs while you stay downstairs (for 5, 10, 15, and 30 minutes, then for 1 hour).
	Mom goes into other rooms without singing to you.
(bottom)	You stay in living room while Mom is in kitchen (for 5, 10, 15, 20, and 30 minutes).

Thelma practiced her relaxation and deep breathing, read her self-talk note cards, studied the thinking mistakes that she made and how to think more correct or realistic thoughts, and used her tools to master her worry. When she was ready, Thelma took the first step on her ladder: to go in the living room while her mom was in the nearby kitchen. She started slow, doing it for 5 minutes, then did it for longer periods of time—10, 15, 20, and 30 minutes—eventually being able to be in the living room alone for more than an hour! It wasn't easy, but it wasn't nearly as hard as she thought it would be. The first time she did it, she called to her mom, who popped her head in the living room and told Thelma that she was facing her fears and doing a fantastic job. She did it again and again, and then it became very easy, and did not cause her to feel scared or nervous at all. By the third time, she did not have to ask her mom to come in, and she learned to feel comfortable being in the living room alone. She was able to relax and enjoy watching TV and reading a book. Then Thelma felt ready to take the second step: her mother would go into other rooms in the house while Thelma was in the living room or her bedroom, but her mom would not sing to her. Again, she felt nervous and scared the first time they practiced, but it got easier and easier with each practice, and soon Thelma did not feel nervous when her mother left the room. Thelma remembered to do her breathing and read her self-talk note cards. She also told herself that feeling nervous was normal, but that it would get better, and it did.

Your child is told that like Thelma, she will build a ladder and team to help her face her fears. Looking at Thelma's ladder will help your child do this.

To be part of your child's team, you'll have to identify what you need to do to make the steps on the ladder go smoothly. As described above, Thelma's mom did many things to help Thelma to not feel anxious, including:

- ▶ Singing to Thelma as she went in different rooms in the house.
- ▶ Allowing Thelma to sleep with her in her bed.
- ▶ Avoid leaving the house without her as much as possible.

These behaviors served to accommodate Thelma's anxiety. Unfortunately, such behaviors tend to make anxiety worse. Loving, caring, warm parents want to put their child at ease and make the anxiety lessen. Loving, caring, warm parents end up unintentionally reinforcing the anxiety by accommodating it and by providing their child with reassurance. It gives the child the message that her anxiety *is* that bad—it's so bad that it's worth addressing and focusing on and even changing the way we live. You know better than anyone what it's like for your child to turn to you to make everything OK. This may come out in the form of questions, such as, "What will we be doing tomorrow?" and "Will you definitely be home in an hour?" and "You still love me, right?" or it may come out in behavior, such as when your child throws a tantrum if he or she isn't allowed to sleep in bed with you. In an effort to soothe your child and make it better, you give into these demands—you answer the questions, you avoid doing things that are hard for your child to handle. The most wonderful parents do this instinctively. The funny thing is, it doesn't work. It provides temporary relief at best. Your child likely asks these questions repetitively, but the answers do not solve the worry or lessen the anxiety.

You are the instrumental part of your child's team in facing his fears. As such an important team member, it is essential that your role entails being supportive and encouraging, but *not* accommodating. For example, Thelma's mother needed to learn that she had to stop singing as she went in different rooms, could not allow Thelma to sleep with her (nor sleep with Thelma in Thelma's room), and could not stay at home to avoid prompting a meltdown. Her mother stopped giving these accommodations in a gradual way so as not to overwhelm Thelma. Once Thelma endorsed that she was ready to face her fears, her mom would meet her at that goal. For instance, once Thelma felt ready to have her mother leave the room without singing to her, Thelma's mother had to stop singing, even if during the exposure, Thelma got upset or requested that her mom sing. In sum, you will stop accommodating your child's anxiety in a step-by-step fashion, as she takes the steps on her ladder, but you will need to be firm and consistent by not giving in. At times it will be quite challenging and possibly very upsetting to you; however, it is necessary to end these accommodations in order for your child to become anxiety-free. Don't forget that one of the ways that you can help your child deal with not having you accommodate his anxiety is to comment on the process: "I know this is hard for you, and it's hard for me, too. A part of me wants to sing to you because I know it will make you feel better in that moment, but it will make the anxiety worse overall. It will make the anxiety bigger and stronger, and as a team, we need to fight it by not giving in. It will get easier with practice." Also, remind your child to use his tools by saying, "What can you do right now to help yourself feel better?" If he does not know, remind him of the strategies he can use: breathing, self-talk, conquer worry strategies, and so on.

The exercise for this chapter involves creating your child's team and the ladder (the hierarchy of anxiety-provoking situations). I deliberately placed the exercise of creating the hierarchy as one of the earliest projects because it frames the goals that your child is working toward. Below are two additional sample ladders and brief descriptions of the exposure process. Reviewing these will help you better understand the process of making the ladder and ordering the steps from least to most anxiety-producing.

Sample 1: James (Snake Phobia)

Taking Steps With Snakes

(top)	Be near a live snake out of his cage up close (within 6 inches).
	Be near a live snake out of his cage from a distance (2 feet away).
	Be near a live snake in his cage up close (within 6 inches).
	Be near a live snake in his cage from a distance (2 feet away).
	Touch a snakeskin.
	Standing near a bush (and when it is rustled by an animal).
	Watching a video with snakes.
	Hearing the sounds of a snake (hissing sound).
	Looking at pictures of snakes.
	Reading about snakes.
(bottom)	Talking about snakes.

James and I made his ladder together and he was very involved in planning the exposures. For example, he went to the library and checked out books on snakes and movies with snake scenes. We watched a scene from *The Black Stallion* in which the boy in the movie had a terrifying encounter with a cobra snake, watched an informational video on how to care for your pet snake (not that James's goals included having a pet snake!), and watched the scene from the *Harry Potter* movie that included an animated snake. When it came time to be near live snakes, James and I started with a trip to the National Zoo's Reptile House. At first, he kept his distance, but on our second visit, he felt comfortable enough to go close up to the glass enclosure. We went to the pet store three times together, and each time he got closer and closer to the live snake (we requested that the snake be taken out of the cage). James and I laughed about the fact that the same employee helped us every time, but had no idea what we were doing there. We could tell by the third visit that she thought it was a little strange that we wanted to see the snake, but not too close, and certainly did not want to touch or hold it (of course, the assumption in a pet store is that we would be interested in buying a snake). I told James that it's our right to go into the pet store, without buying (or even handling) the pet snakes! After our last trip to the pet store, I took James to an ice cream shop for an ice cream treat. He enjoyed this reward immensely and felt proud of himself for all of his hard work on facing his fears. Eventually, he visited the house of his friend with the pet snake. James attended a total of 12 sessions of CBT with me, and by the end, he no longer met the criteria for a snake phobia. His parents commented that James seemed happier and more confident in himself.

Sample 2: Ruth (OCD)

Getting Over Germs!

(top)	Using a public bathroom and rewearing your clothes the next day.
	Using a public bathroom and washing your clothes only once afterward.
	Touching the door on the way out of the public bathroom with your hands.

	Touching the faucet in a public bathroom with your hands.
	Touching the stall door lock and handle of a public bathroom with your hands.
	Flushing the toilet in a public bathroom using your hands.
	Using a public bathroom and touching the door on the way in with your hands.
	Using a public bathroom.
	Eating from the school cafeteria.
	Eating homemade cookies and brownies.
	Eating from a "shared" bowl in a public place.
	Eating from a "shared" bowl at a party.
(bottom)	Eating at home with an "unclean" utensil (hand-washed only).

Ruth's treatment involved a lot of education. First of all, she needed to understand that germs are neither dangerous nor threatening. She learned that we are exposed to germs every day and that we need germs to be healthy (I explained, in detail, that our bodies make special things called *antibodies* that prevent us from getting sick and that the only way our bodies can make these special antibodies is to be exposed to germs). Ruth also learned that germs are all over everything, a part of our environment, and that we cannot see germs. I emphasized that I was not trying to make her more anxious; rather, I was helping her understand that germs are a normal part of life. I explained the difference between being hygienic (washing our hands after using the bathroom and before and after meals, washing our clothes) and being irrational (refusing to eat from a bowl of chips at a party). I assured her that taking the steps on her ladder would not make her sick, and I modeled these steps for her. In one session, I literally took some chips and put them on the floor, then picked them up and ate them. She looked disgusted with me as I did this, but I told her I was doing something extreme to show her that nothing bad would happen. I reassured her the next week that I did not get sick from eating the chips, and in fact, they tasted just as good as if I'd eaten them from the bag. I also assured her that I do not make it a habit of eating off of the floor.

Facing one's fear is at the core of cognitive-behavioral treatment for anxiety disorders. Up until now, your child has likely been accommodating her anxiety, living her life avoiding those situations that cause her to feel nervous, uncomfortable, and scared. By forming a "team" and "team goals," you are helping your child begin to take back control in her life, and to overcome her anxiety and fears. The next chapter will focus on learning how to relax and calm the body.

Chapter 2 Exercise

Tips for Parents

1. Because forming the hierarchy involves listing many or all of your child's fear situations, he may feel a little overwhelmed (or anxious) about the prospect of having to complete the situations on his ladder. This is why it is crucial for you to remind your child of two things:

    a. Your child will not have to face his fears just yet; first, he will learn many tools and strategies to manage the task of facing fears.

    b. Your child will not be forced to face his fears. Rather, your child will go at his own pace. Although you will encourage your child, you will not force him to face his fears.

2. When developing the list of anxiety-provoking situations for your child, you may want to ask yourself the following questions: What things are hard for your child to do because he is anxious about doing them? What things do you avoid doing because they are upsetting/anxiety-provoking to your child? What are other children you know capable of doing that your child is not (e.g., riding a bike, going on a play date)? You also may want to ask extended family members or your closest friends what they observe to be challenging for your child to do because of his anxiety and include these situations in the ladder.

3. Remember to be very encouraging with your child as the two of you complete the ladder. You want to make it as positive and fun as possible, and ensure that it is not a shaming experience for him. Some children are sensitive about listing the many different things that are hard for them to do. If your child begins to feel this way, or expresses embarrassment about his anxiety, then remind

him of how common it is: that many children have anxiety. Tell him, "It's the most common problem for kids, and 1 out of 10 children have problems with anxiety." It is essential that you do not allow his embarrassment to prevent you from doing the exercise; is it possible that your child may be magnifying the embarrassment as a way to avoid facing his fears. In this case, label it as resistance and talk with your child (in a calm, nonblaming tone) about his concerns about treating the anxiety. Also, tell him how proud you are of him; provide positive reinforcement like praise and reward ("Let's do this and then watch your favorite movie").

4. As recommended below, I always leave a few spaces between some of the steps just in case you and your child decide to add some more situations (this often occurs once you have begun the exposure process).

5. When doing the exposures on their ladder, children will find it helpful if you can model for them first. So, if your child has social anxiety and she worries about sending food back in a restaurant or spilling something in public, show her it's not so bad by first doing it yourself. This also will help her feel more confident about being able to do the exposures.

6. Finally, it is ideal if you can make the ladder as specific as possible, including the duration of the exposure, starting out small and gradually making it longer. For example, Thelma started out with her mom in the kitchen while she was in the living room alone for 5 minutes and gradually made it up to 30 minutes.

Exercises

Making Your Team and Team Goals

WHO IS ON YOUR TEAM?

Write in the names of the members of your team in the blanks below. You do not have to fill in all of the blanks. Your team will be at least three people: You (the captain), whoever is reading the parent book (usually mom or dad), and me (Dr. Zucker). Other people you can include on your team are your grandparents, sister or brother, babysitter or nanny, pets, and your therapist if you have one. Your team members all will help you to face your fears in different ways. For example, Thelma's dog, Sniffy, was on her team and Sniffy helped her face her fears by being with her in the beginning when she was nervous about her Mom leaving her alone in the living room. Sniffy also gave her extra licks when she was happy about doing such a great job in facing her fears.

YOUR TEAM:

1. Team Captain: _____
                              (your name here)
2. _____
3. _____
4. _____
5. _____
6. _____

Team Goals: Making Your Ladder

You will need the following materials to make your ladder:

▶ Blank note cards
▶ Poster board (white or another light color)
▶ Markers
▶ Pen or pencil
▶ Stickers (stars, happy faces, whatever you want)

TO MAKE YOUR LADDER:

1. Using note cards and a pen or pencil, write down all of the different things that are hard for you to do or that you avoid doing because of anxiety and worry. Your mom or dad (or both) will help you make this list. Write each of these things on a different note card (sometimes kids and their parents choose to write it down on a piece of paper before they write it on the note cards; either way works, just as long as each thing is written on a note card).

2. Use the floor or a table and spread out all of the note cards. Then look carefully at each of the note cards and put them in order from easiest to hardest (your parent will help). The easiest ones will be on the bottom and the hardest ones will be up at the top. Here is what Thelma's note cards looked like before she made them into a ladder:

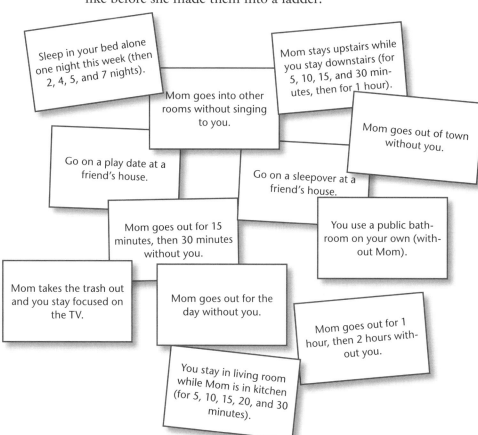

Sleep in your bed alone one night this week (then 2, 4, 5, and 7 nights).

Mom goes into other rooms without singing to you.

Mom stays upstairs while you stay downstairs (for 5, 10, 15, and 30 minutes, then for 1 hour).

Mom goes out of town without you.

Go on a play date at a friend's house.

Go on a sleepover at a friend's house.

Mom goes out for 15 minutes, then 30 minutes without you.

You use a public bathroom on your own (without Mom).

Mom takes the trash out and you stay focused on the TV.

Mom goes out for the day without you.

Mom goes out for 1 hour, then 2 hours without you.

You stay in living room while Mom is in kitchen (for 5, 10, 15, 20, and 30 minutes).

3. Now count your note cards. How many do you have? _____

4. Come up with a title for your ladder. Write the name here:

_____

Now, write the title at the top of the poster board.

5. Use the poster board and markers to draw a great big ladder with steps, under where you wrote the title. The number of steps you draw should be the same as the number of note cards you have. Leave a little space here and there in between some of the steps, just in case you decide to add more things later on.
6. Write the steps, from easiest to hardest, on the ladder using the markers.

The stickers will be used once you start doing the steps. We won't begin doing this just yet; first you need to learn some tools (or ways) to deal with your anxious feelings and worries. You will first learn how to help the **body** part of anxiety. In the next chapter, you will learn about relaxation and deep breathing.

3

Relaxing the Body

Kimberly started to notice that when she was anxious or worried, her body felt different. Her muscles were tight and tense, her heartbeat would speed up, and she seemed to always have a stomachache or a headache. Kimberly and her mom learned different ways to relax her body, and she started to learn how to loosen her muscles and slow her heartbeat down. Kimberly also liked practicing relaxing imagery with her dad before he tucked her in at night.

THIS chapter focuses on addressing the physiological or body part of anxiety. In Chapter 1, you and your child learned that the body has a reaction when you feel anxious. In this chapter, you and your child will learn how to do the three types of relaxation:

1. Calm Breathing,
2. Progressive Muscle Relaxation (PMR), and
3. Relaxing Imagery.

Learning how to relax should be a positive experience for your child, so try to frame it that way when the two of you complete the exercise at the end. The goal is for your child to become a master of relaxation. Because it is physiologically impossible to be relaxed and anxious at the same time, if your child uses his relaxation skills at the time he feels anxious, he will not be anxious any more.

The following sections include scripts for you to use with your child to help her relax.

Calm Breathing

Breathing in a calm, relaxed way means that you are breathing in through your nose and out through your mouth, and the air is going all the way down to the lowest part of your belly. This is the opposite from breathing in an anxious, tense way when your breathing is shallow and the air only goes down as far as the upper part of your chest.

Have your child try doing this: *Breathe in through your nose for 4 seconds and then out through your mouth for 4 seconds.* As she does this, have her try to get the air that she breathes in to go all the way to the bottom of her belly, below her belly button. It helps to have her put her hands on this part of her abdomen and then try to get her hands to move up and down as she breathes in and out. Encourage her to try not to let any air stop, or get stuck, in the top of her chest; tell her to just let the air go in easily through her nose all of the way to the bottom of her belly.

Look at Thelma as she learns how to do calm breathing. Notice how her lower belly goes out as she breathes in.

Say the following to your child: *"Breathe in through your nose for 4 seconds, hold the breath for 4 seconds, and then slowly breathe out through your mouth for 4 seconds."* It also may help if she practices doing this when lying down. This way she can look at the bottom of her belly and make it rise up when she breathes in and fall down when she breathes out.

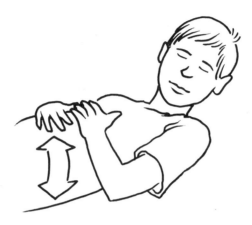

Sometimes kids will have a hard time catching their breath when they are anxious. If this happens, have her try breathing in and out through only one nostril. Say the following to your child: *"Hold one of your nostrils closed and close your mouth, and breathe in and out through the one open nostril."* It will help if the two of you practice together; this way you can model the pacing for her, showing her how to take long, slow breaths in and out through only one nostril.

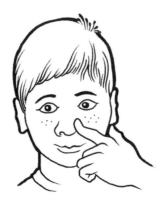

Progressive Muscle Relaxation (PMR)

PMR is a type of relaxation that involves making your muscles relax by first tightening them up and holding them for about 5–10 seconds. Your child will do one section of the body at a time, starting with his hands and going all the way down to his feet. When your child does PMR, try to have him focus on what it feels like when his muscles are tight and tense and when they are loose and relaxed. Here is a script for you and your child to use to practice PMR:

1. Start by making tight fists, imagining that you are squeezing the juice out of a lemon. Hold your fists nice and tight and count to 10. Then let go and shake it out (shake your hands out).

2. Now pull your arms into your body next to your ribs. Tighten up your bicep and forearms muscles, but do not make fists or tighten your hands. Hold it for 1, 2, 3, 4, 5, 6, 7, 8, 9, and 10 then let it go and shake it out. Remember to notice what your muscles feel like when they are tense and when they are loose. Sometimes once you loosen them, your muscles will feel a little tingly.

3. Bring your shoulders all the way up toward your ears and tighten them up; this also should make the back of your neck tight. Hold it for the count of 10 then allow your shoulders to drop down toward your hips. As you do this, say the word relax to yourself and also breathe out slowly through your mouth.

4. Now pull your shoulders back and arch your back in toward your chest. Imagine that there is a string connected to your chest and someone is pulling the string up, lifting your chest up toward the ceiling. This will tighten your back. Hold it for 10 then let it go and feel the difference between tension and relaxation.

5. Squeeze and pull your stomach, or abdominal, muscles in toward your spine. Keep it tight for 10 seconds then let it go.

6. Now squeeze your buttocks muscles (they are important, too!), and hold for 10 seconds then let go and loosen them up.

7. Stick your legs and feet straight out in front of you and point your toes in toward your chest. This will tighten the muscles in your legs and thighs. Make the muscles as tight as you can and hold for 10 seconds, then let go and allow your legs to gently drop to the ground and relax.

8. Stick your legs and feet straight out in front of you again, but this time point your toes straight out away from you and tighten up the muscles in your legs, thighs, and feet. Try to get it so you feel a little cramping in the bottom of your feet. Hold for 10 seconds then let go, allowing your legs to gently drop to the floor.

9. Now we will tighten up all of the muscles in your face. Start by clenching your teeth and jaw. Then squish up your nose, lifting it up, and close your eyes and squeeze the muscles around them, and tighten up your forehead. Hold this tightness in your whole face for 10 seconds then let go and relax. Open your mouth a little bit and move your jaw from left to right and then in circles. This will allow the jaw to become even more relaxed.

10. Last step: WHOLE BODY! You want to go from being a stiff, tight **robot** to being a loose, relaxed **rag doll**! Start with tight fists, then add arms, bring shoulders up to your ears and then pull them back to tighten your back, squeeze your stomach into your spine, tighten your buttocks, put your legs out in front of you with your toes pointing out away from you and cramp up your feet, and tighten your jaw and whole face. HOLD FOR 10 SECONDS (ROBOT) and then LET GO (RAG DOLL), loosening every muscle in your body. I could tell if you were a really relaxed rag doll if I tried to lift up your arm and it felt very heavy and loose.

Relaxing Imagery

Relaxing imagery is another type of relaxation, and it is best to first learn and practice it at home or in your therapist's office. This type of relaxation offers your child the opportunity to become deeply relaxed and really "let go" of tension and stress. You will guide your child in a guided relaxation as part of the exercise at the end of this chapter.

When preparing to practice, encourage your child to find a comfortable place to sit or lie down. Some kids really like to use pillows, too. If she wants to use pillows to get more comfortable, have her try putting one under her head, another one under her knees, and she may like putting one under each of her arms. You and your child may enjoy listening to some relaxing music (with no words) in the background. Here is a script for you to use with your child to teach her about relaxing imagery:

Once you are comfortable, I want you to **close your eyes and take a deep breath in through your nose and out through your mouth**. As you breathe in, imagine that you are breathing in clean, relaxing air and as you breathe out, let go of any stress or tension that you are holding onto. Breathing in, you let calm air go all the way down to the bottom of your belly. Breathing out, you let go of the air and your belly becomes flat. With each breath, you feel more and more relaxed.

Imagine that you are standing in a hallway. This is the most beautiful hallway you have ever been in—the floor is cushiony and soft, and the colors that surround you are all of your favorites. The temperature is perfect—cool but not too cool and you feel a slight breeze on your face. You notice that your body begins to loosen up.

You begin to walk down the hallway and as you do, you feel lighter and lighter. The hallway curves around to the left and then curves around to the right. As you are walking, you see that it is getting brighter and brighter, and then the hallway ends in a beautiful room.

This room is filled with windows, several of which are cracked open just a bit, allowing a nice, cool, refreshing breeze to flow through the room. Sunlight is streaming in through the windows. You walk into the room and there is a big, soft, fluffy couch up against the wall. You decide to sit and then lie down on the couch. Your body is completely supported by the couch and there is a large, fluffy pillow under your head, and another one under your knees, taking away any tension from your neck and shoulders and back and feet.

As you lie there you feel the sunlight on your body, covering you from head to toe, warming you, and you feel the cool breeze flowing over you. The combination of the warm sun and the cool breeze makes you feel even more relaxed, and you begin to fall into a deep state of relaxation. You remind yourself this is your time for relaxation.

You have nowhere to go and nothing to do. Any thoughts that come into your mind simply flow in and flow out. You don't need to hold onto any thoughts—just let them flow by.

Just outside this room, there are some orange and grapefruit trees. This is a very safe, very relaxing place. Just past the trees is a beach. You begin to think about this beach and the ocean. You imagine yourself standing at the shoreline and can feel the wet sand as it goes in between your toes. You look out into the crystal clear water and see that there are the most beautiful fish swimming by. You look at the fish—they are all different colors—purple, turquoise, yellow, and black, and then you see a few starfish on the ocean floor. Then some beautiful stingrays swim by—you like to watch as the water changes the shape of their bodies. You are very relaxed as you watch these fish.

Then you focus on the waves, and watch as they come into the shore and then go out back into the ocean. Flowing in and then flowing out and then just flowing along. Nature is very peaceful.

Lying back on the couch, you think more about these waves. In just a moment, you will imagine a wave coming over your body, and as it does, it will soothe and comfort you, and then it will slowly leave your body, taking away any remaining tension and tightness. The wave can be any color—blue, green, purple—or it can be clear. Imagine the wave slowly going over your toes, feet, and ankles. Then it goes up your legs, knees, and thighs. It goes over your hips, hands, arms, and stomach, all the way up to your shoulders, but not over your neck. The wave is warm and comforting. It hangs out for just a minute, relaxing and soothing all of your muscles. Then the wave begins to leave, taking away all remaining tension, going down your stomach, arms, hands, and hips; all the way down past your thighs, knees, legs, and ankles; and then finally leaves your feet and toes. You are now even more relaxed.

Take a moment to enjoy this relaxation, noticing how calm and slow your breathing is. In just a minute, count to 10, and imagine yourself climbing up a set of stairs. With each step, you become more and more alert, but still very relaxed. At the top of the stairs, there will be an archway. You will walk through the archway and then you will be back in your own room, taking with you all the feelings of relaxation.

One, take the first step.
Two, take the second step.
Three, take the third step.

Four, take the fourth step.
Five, take the fifth step.
Six, take the sixth step,
Seven, take the seventh step.
Eight, take the eighth step.
Nine, take the ninth step.
And ten, take the tenth step.

Walk through the archway, and you are back in your room. Remind yourself that you can become this relaxed anytime you'd like, and it will only take 5 minutes!

You and your child can practice relaxing imagery with this scene or with any other relaxing scene. Below are a few additional scenes that are not included in your child's book. You can use these scenes when helping your child practice relaxing imagery. When reading the scene, try to use a calm and soft voice; you may choose to play background music (without words) on a low volume. Your child also is encouraged to come up with his own mental picture of a relaxing scene, which can be a real or an imaginary place.

Alternative Scene #1: Forest Scene

This scene begins the same as the scene above, but involves going to the forest, rather than the beach:

Once you are comfortable, I want you to **close your eyes and take a deep breath in through your nose and out through your mouth.** As you breathe in, imagine that you are breathing in clean, relaxing air and as you breathe out, let go of any stress or tension that you are holding onto. Breathing in, you let calm air go all the way down to the bottom of your belly. Breathing out, you let go of the air and your belly becomes flat. With each breath, you feel more and more relaxed.

Imagine that you are standing in a hallway. This is the most beautiful hallway you have ever been in—the floor is cushiony and soft, and the colors that surround you are all of your favorites. The temperature is perfect—cool but not too cool and you feel a slight breeze on your face. You notice that your body begins to loosen up.

You begin to walk down the hallway and as you do, you feel lighter and lighter. The hallway curves around to the left and then curves around to the right. As you are walking, you see that it is getting brighter and brighter, and then the hallway ends in a magical forest. This forest is the most beautiful and serene place you have ever been. The floor on which you stand is soft and as you take a few steps, you hear the crackling sound of the leaves that you step on. You look all the way up to the sky and you see the tops of the tall trees and you notice that the sun is streaming in through the leaves at the top of these trees. On the forest floor, there are spots of sunlight and this creates a warm feeling inside of you. There is a slight breeze and you can smell the pine in the air. As you gently walk through the forest, you see a stream ahead and you decide to go near it. You let your fingers gently touch the water as it glides over the rocks in the stream. Just down the stream are two deer drinking from its cool water. You notice that your body feels calm and light and you are free from any thoughts. You are just focused on being in the forest and feeling very, very relaxed.

You continue to walk in the forest and see a soft patch of green grass. You decide to sit and then lie down on the green grass. Lying on your back, you look up at the sky again and see the tops of the trees sway from left to right and right to left. The wind is blowing the leaves and branches around, and you love to hear the sound of the wind as it blows. Feeling so calm and so relaxed, you decide to gently close your eyes. You continue to hear the sounds of the forest and feel the warmth of the sun and the coolness of the slight breeze. You are very, very relaxed and very safe. Take some time to enjoy this relaxed feeling. If you notice any part of your body that feels tight, just imagine that part loosening up, and tell the muscle to "let go." Notice how calm and slow your breathing is.

In just a minute, I will count to 10, and I want you to imagine yourself climbing up a set of stairs. With each step, you become more and more alert, but still very relaxed. At the top of the stairs, there will be an archway. You will walk through the archway and then you will be back in your own room, taking with you all the feelings of relaxation.

One, take the first step.
Two, take the second step.
Three, take the third step.
Four, take the fourth step.
Five, take the fifth step.

Six, take the sixth step,
Seven, take the seventh step.
Eight, take the eighth step.
Nine, take the ninth step.
And ten, take the tenth step.

Walk through the archway and gently open your eyes. You are back in your own room. Remind yourself that you can become this relaxed anytime you'd like, and it will only take 5 minutes!

Alternative Scene #2: Raft Scene

This scene can either be used in lieu of the relaxation scene in your child's book, or in addition to it (when he is standing at the beach, before he returns to lying on the couch). If you are using it in lieu of the one in his book, it will begin the same way.

Once you are comfortable, I want you to **close your eyes and take a deep breath in through your nose and out through your mouth**. As you breathe in, imagine that you are breathing in clean, relaxing air and as you breathe out, let go of any stress or tension that you are holding onto. Breathing in, you let calm air go all the way down to the bottom of your belly. Breathing out, you let go of the air and your belly becomes flat. With each breath, you feel more and more relaxed.

Imagine that you are standing in a hallway. This is the most beautiful hallway you have ever been in—the floor is cushiony and soft, and the colors that surround you are all of your favorites. The temperature is perfect—cool but not too cool and you feel a slight breeze on your face. You notice that your body begins to loosen up.

You begin to walk down the hallway and as you do, you feel lighter and lighter. The hallway curves around to the left and then curves around to the right. As you are walking, you see that it is getting brighter and brighter, and then the hallway ends in at a beautiful beach. This is the most beautiful beach you have ever seen. The sand is perfectly white and soft, and not too hot. The water is crystal clear and perfectly turquoise in color. You walk toward the shoreline and look out into ocean. You can smell the salt in the air and hear the sound of the water as it gently hits the land. There are very few waves; the water is very calm. In front of you is a big, fully inflated raft. This raft is very special because it has a secret window on the bottom of it that lets you clearly see what's in the ocean. You decide to give the raft a push into the water and you get on it. Immediately, you feel wonderful. You love the feeling of floating on the water. The raft is plush and very comfortable. First, you lie on your back and feel the water move you along, in a gentle back and forth motion. The sun is warming your body, and you feel very relaxed and very safe. You decide to slowly turn over on your stomach and look through the secret window. Below you is a world full of beautiful sea life. Coral of all different bright colors—orange, pink, and green—lines the ocean floor. You see starfish on some of the coral. Magical fish swim by underneath you— purple, yellow, and pink fish—all different colors. Stingrays glide by and you love to see the shape of their bodies change as they swim in the water. The longer you look, the more relaxed you feel. You are not holding onto any thoughts—you are just being in the moment, and you are very calm. Focus on what you see and how you feel. Your back feels warm and soothed by the sun, and you feel a slight ocean breeze flowing over you. Take a moment to enjoy this feeling of relaxation.

In just a minute, I will count to 10, and I want you to imagine yourself climbing up a set of stairs. With each step, you become more and more alert, but still very relaxed. At the top of the stairs, there will be an archway. You will walk through the archway and then you will be back in your own room, taking with you all the feelings of relaxation.

One, take the first step.
Two, take the second step.
Three, take the third step.
Four, take the fourth step.
Five, take the fifth step.
Six, take the sixth step,
Seven, take the seventh step.
Eight, take the eighth step.
Nine, take the ninth step.
And ten, take the tenth step.

Walk through the archway and gently open your eyes. You are back in your own room. Remind yourself that you can become this relaxed anytime you'd like, and it will only take 5 minutes!

Stress Management

Managing daily stress is essential in reducing overall anxiety and lowering one's baseline. In order to teach your child about stress management, she will learn about the "beaker" analogy. A beaker is used to represent someone's stress level. Everyone always has some fluid in their beaker, which signifies the daily stressors, like forgetting to turn in homework or, for adults, forgetting to pay a bill on time.

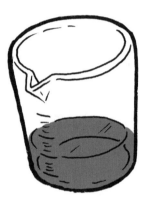

When additional events occur, such as getting a bad grade on a test, or events related to your child's anxiety disorder, the beaker level can go way up.

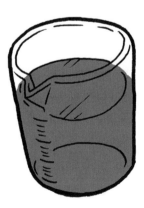

Once someone's beaker is at the top, it only takes something small, *any little thing*, to cause it to overflow. When our beakers overflow, we explode—have a meltdown, scream, yell, panic, and cry, whatever. It's up to your child to lower his own beaker level (and it is up to you, the parent, to monitor yours). Though you may help your child feel better at times, you want to encourage your child to take responsibility for his emotions—this promotes the skill of self-regulation, or learning how to manage his reaction to different events.

Here are some ideas on what your child can do to lower his beaker level:

1. Sleep well.
2. Eat well.
3. Exercise.
4. Do relaxation.
5. Express his feelings appropriately.
6. Take a hot bath, and add bubbles if he likes (but not too hot).
7. Do 100 jumping jacks or push-ups (after that she'll feel too exhausted to be stressed!).
8. Write in a journal—write about what is bothering him and what he can do to make it better.
9. Paint a picture or do an art project.
10. Play an instrument.
11. Play with a pet (dog, cat).
12. Call a friend.
13. Distract herself by reading a book or watching TV or a movie.
14. Ask someone to help her cook something.
15. Play outside.

Your child's book encourages your child to come up with additional ways that personally help him to feel better and less anxious. I am a big fan of yoga, and find that it has made an enormous difference in my ability to manage stress (and lowering my "baseline," making it much easier for me to handle things when they come my way). I practice the Iyengar method, which focuses on facilitating alignment and strength; there are many different types of yoga to try. In my work with children with anxiety, I often teach them a few yoga moves and the majority of them show a great interest in learning about it.

In your child's book, space is allotted for him to write down other ways that he can lower his beaker level. Because the exercise at the end of this chapter in your child's book involves a discussion on how you, his parent, manages stress, write down *your* ideas on how you can lower *your own* beaker on the lines below:

_____

_____

_____

_____

_____

_____

_____

_____

_____

Finally, it is important that your child stays on top of school-work and other extracurricular demands, as this is helpful in reducing worry associated with getting everything done. I also rec-ommend that children *and adults* have one day each week that is free from doing *any* schoolwork (or work), because everyone needs a break and one day each week that focuses on relaxing and have fun. Nurturing your child's social needs also is recommended.

Chapter 3 Exercise

Tips for Parents

1. The exercise below includes a discussion topic for you and your child. You will need to be prepared to share ways in which you personally manage your own stress, and what you do to relax and calm down. Try to generate examples that your child can relate to, such as lying in the sun, going to the zoo, and so forth.

2. When helping your child practice relaxation, try to create the right environment for your child to feel comfortable. For example, find a space in your home (or outside) where there is minimal or no noise, where the temperature is neutral, and where your child can really relax. Some parents have made a ritual out of it for their child: dimming the lights, lighting candles, and lying on blankets or mats on the floor. The best part is this will offer an opportunity for you to relax as well!

Practice Relaxation

Your exercise this week includes:

1. A topic question for you and your mom or dad to talk about.
2. Making a calm breathing note card.
3. Practicing your relaxation 5 days this week.

Try not to think of practicing the relaxation as a chore, but as something that feels very good that you can look forward to doing. Knowing how to relax is one of the most important tools you will use when we get to the "facing your fears" part. Your mom or dad will help you by practicing with you over the week.

DISCUSSION TOPIC

Talk to your mom or dad about what makes them feel relaxed—what they do to calm down and manage stress. Tell your mom or dad what makes you feel relaxed and what you think can help you calm down. Your mom or dad might want to know what they can do to help you feel less stressed.

1. Use one note card to write down how to do calm breathing. Make your note card look like this one:

Calm Breathing

In → nose → 4 seconds
Hold → 4 seconds
Out → mouth → 4 seconds

Then on the back, make yours look like this:

Calm Breathing

Breathe in and out through only one nostril. Hold your other nostril closed and close your mouth.

---

2. Practice relaxation! Check off the days that you practiced and what type of relaxation you did in the chart below:

Day of the Week	Calm Breathing	Progressive Muscle Relaxation (PMR)	Relaxing Imagery
Monday			
Tuesday			
Wednesday			
Thursday			
Friday			
Saturday			
Sunday			

Exercises

4

Conquer
Your Worries

"What if I can't finish all of this homework? There is so much to do. I don't even know where to start. There is no way I will finish," thought Kimberly when she sat down to do her homework. She also worried about break-ins, being kidnapped, and her dog escaping. Kimberly's mom helped her make a list of her worries, and Kimberly realized that they were the same worries almost every day. She scheduled "worry time" and soon she started to worry less overall. She began to label her worries as "anxiety" and started to talk back to them. Kimberly's mom also helped her learn that the anticipatory anxiety was not a good predictor of what was to come.

"When I think back on all these worries, I remember the story of the old man who said on his deathbed that he had a lot of trouble in his life, most of which never happened."

—Winston Churchill

IN this chapter, you and your child will learn how to get rid of worries. Worries are thoughts (this chapter and Chapter 5 are about the "thoughts" part of anxiety), and as the quote above illustrates, most worries are a waste of time. Worry breeds self-doubt, which can cause a negative impact on your child's self-esteem, especially if the worrying is chronic. This chapter will help your child learn how to deal with his worries and ultimately to feel more confident. A primary goal of this program is to promote a sense of empowerment in your child; this will be accomplished largely by having your child face his fears.

There are six parts of conquering worry (each of these are covered in your child's book):

1. understanding the two types of worry and asking two important questions,
2. getting the big picture,
3. scheduling "worry time,"
4. positive self-talk,
5. talking back to the anxiety, and
6. dealing with anticipatory anxiety.

Understanding the Two Types of Worry: Useful and Useless Worry

One way to challenge worries is to differentiate between those that are useful or helpful and those that are useless. As you probably know, some amount of anxiety is often beneficial, as it motivates you to get things done in a timely manner. **Useful** worry, therefore, helps you be more productive without causing a negative physiological reaction (e.g., rapid heart rate, tight muscles, upset stomach). **Useless** worry is worry that causes an interruption, or impairment, in your ability to get things done. In fact, this type of worry often can prevent you from being productive and often results in a negative physiological reaction (e.g., rapid heart rate, tight muscles, upset stomach).

In your child's book, she will learn to label useless worry as "just the anxiety talking," and the exercise at the end of this chapter is designed to help her with this process. Through facing her fears, your child will learn that there was nothing to worry about in the first place, confirming that her worry was useless. She also will learn that worrying makes her feel a false sense of control. It does this by making her feel like she is doing something to deal with her anxiety (i.e., worrying). In fact, just the opposite is true—worrying actually strengthens her anxiety about the situation and makes the event seem worse.

Asking Yourself Two Things

When you are worried, ask yourself the following two questions:
(1) What is the worst thing that could happen?
(2) Could I handle it?

The answer is *always* "yes." Remind your child that he can handle anything that comes his way, and that you can handle anything that comes your way. Reinforce that although bad things can happen, there is nothing in life that he cannot handle.

Big Picture Perspective

When you are worried, try to get the "big picture" perspective by asking yourself the following:

"At the end of your very, very long and very, very wonderful life, will it really matter if _____?
Will this really matter in the big picture?"
(Fill in what you are worried about.)

For example, if your child is worried about a math test coming up and this worry interferes with his ability to fall asleep, encourage him to adopt the big picture outlook and ask himself:

"At the end of my very, very long and very, very wonderful life, will it really matter if <u>I didn't do well on this one math test in fifth grade</u>?"

The truth is that in the big picture of life, it really won't matter if he didn't do well on this one test in one subject during one semester of school. Although it is important that your child try his best at school, this technique is used to help him get a grip on his excessive anxiety (e.g., anxiety that is causing an impairment, such as insomnia) about the math test. The purpose is to help him manage his anxiety about the test, which may even improve his performance on it.

Perhaps your child becomes very anxious about going to a birthday party. Maybe he believes that he will be uncomfortable because he won't know many of the other kids attending; maybe he is having separation anxiety. Encourage him to adopt the "big picture" perspective by asking himself, "In the big picture of life, will it really matter if I went to this one birthday party and didn't have much fun and didn't feel very comfortable?" The truth of the matter is in that in the "big picture" it really won't matter if he didn't have a good time at this one birthday party. However, he needs to go because it is very likely that he will have a lot of fun and could possibly make new friends. Most importantly, going to the party means that he is facing his fears and overcoming his anxiety. The importance of this should not be overlooked or minimized. If your child is in the habit of avoiding situations that he perceives as anxiety-provoking, he likely will continue this pattern over time and ultimately have a very limited comfort zone. He may become increasingly inflexible and self-doubting. The following is an excerpt from the book *One Day My Soul Just Opened Up* by Iyanla Vanzant (1998):

Fear mastered me. It dictated my movements and responses in any given situation. Fear has disguised itself as what I could not do, did not have, and did not have time to do, and as what others would not let me do. I have disguised fear as the need to be somewhere else, doing something else, not knowing how to do something, and not needing to do something. I set a table in my life for fear to become a gluttonous and insatiable master. (p. 214)

Adopting this kind of attitude can result in a very different version of life for your child. But, overcoming his fears can give him a sense of confidence that he never had before, one that could drive him to try new things and embark on great adventures.

Schedule "Worry Time"

Another technique used to conquer worrying is to schedule *worry time* for your child. Worry time consists of setting aside a set amount of time, ranging from 15 minutes to 30 minutes, in which your child intentionally worries. This time is planned out in advance and can be scheduled once or twice a day, depending on how often your child worries (more frequent worrying should involve two worry time sessions). The purpose of this is threefold: first, it helps your child to externalize her worries by "getting them out," but in a structured way versus randomly; second, it helps your child learn to delay worrying until the scheduled time and therefore gives her practice with compartmentalizing her worries; and third, she will begin to see the repetitiveness and uselessness of her worries, as they typically will be the same themes from day to day.

When helping your child structure the worry time, the goal is for her to use the whole time and not stop short. Even if she runs out of things to worry about, she should keep trying to think of things to worry about and if nothing comes up, she should just stay there until the time runs out. This helps create the frame for the worry time and highlights the uselessness of worrying.

There are a few different ways to "worry" during worry time. Your child can choose to simply verbalize her worries or she can write them down like a list. Another option is to record her worries onto an audiocassette tape or a digital voice recorder. If she chooses this option, she can listen to her worries over and over during each worry time (and can use the same recording day after day), and can add onto the tape or voice recorder as she thinks of more worries. Many children with whom I have worked have found the recordings to be extremely useful in getting rid of their worries. The recordings also help desensitize children to their worries, making the worries less meaningful and less powerful.

Positive Self-Talk

Self-talk is what you say to yourself. Children who are anxious often engage in negative self-talk. Some examples include:

"I can't do it."
"I won't be OK."
"I need to be with my mom or dad to feel safe."
"This is too scary."
"I'm too nervous to do this."

When your child tells himself these kinds of things, he strengthens his fears and anxiety. However, if those thoughts are replaced with or challenged by positive self-talk, particularly when your child is being exposed to an anxiety-provoking situation, he will improve his ability to cope and feel more confident about his ability to tolerate the situation. Learning how to tolerate the anxiety-provoking situation is necessary in order for habituation to occur (as mentioned in Chapter 1, habituation is the process of getting used to, or "numbing out" to something; for example, the longer you stay in a freezing cold swimming pool, the warmer the water begins to feel because you have habituated to the temperature).

Here are some examples of positive self-talk:

"I can do it."
"I can handle this."
"Everything is alright."
"I am worried, but I am OK."
"I am anxious, but I can handle it."
"I am scared, but I am safe."
"I can help myself relax."
"I must face my fears to overcome them."
"It is my choice to be calm or be nervous. I am choosing to be
    calm. Let me start by calming my breath."
"It is just the anxiety talking; I don't have to listen to it."

Many kids will use positive self-talk, even though they don't initially believe what they are telling themselves. But with practice, your child will see that these statements are true! The more he uses positive self-talk, the more he will feel like he can handle situations that make him feel anxious.

Talking Back to the Anxiety

Part of self-talk is learning how to "talk back" to the anxiety. By doing this, your child externalizes the anxiety. Externalizing the anxiety allows your child to see the anxiety as something separate from her. This process of externalization enables your child to (1) identify her anxious thoughts and feelings more accurately, (2) challenge these thoughts and feelings and adopt a more balanced way of judging and thinking about anxiety-provoking situations, and (3) face her fears. It is important that your child realize that she and the anxiety are not the same; that the anxiety is a separate thing, even though it often feels like it is part of her. In your child's book, she is told to think of the anxiety as external, or outside of her, something separate. When she has a scary thought, she should say to herself, "It is just the anxiety talking" and remind herself that she doesn't need to listen to it.

The best way for you to help your child deal with useless worries is to encourage her to label them as a *useless worry* and remind her that it is "just the anxiety talking." Emphasize that if she listens to these worries, the anxiety will become stronger and it will win, but if she doesn't listen to it, *she* will become stronger and *she* will win.

Dealing With Anticipatory Anxiety

Anticipatory anxiety is when you feel nervous or worried about something before it actually happens. For example, you tell your child that you will be going out of town for the weekend, and she becomes extremely upset and worried at that moment when you tell her. Maybe she will ask you numerous questions about your plans, or maybe she'll begin to cry and protest your trip. This is called *anticipatory anxiety*, because she is anticipating (or waiting for) something to happen that she perceives as scary. Most anxiety is, in fact, just anticipatory anxiety. Most children end up realizing that their perceived catastrophe was not that bad after all, or that it was difficult at first but then became more comfortable for them (due to habituation). Worrying is about what they fear is *going* to happen, not something that already has happened!

As explained in your child's book, here are the three steps he should learn in order to deal or cope with anticipatory anxiety:

1. Label your worries and scary feelings as "Anticipatory Anxiety." Say to yourself, "It is just anticipatory anxiety."
2. Remind yourself that the thing you are worried about is not going to be as bad as you think or expect it will be. Remind

yourself that the anticipatory anxiety does not make you any more prepared for dealing with the situation you are worried about. Remember, worrying makes you feel a fake sense of control—it makes you feel like you are doing something to deal with the scary situation, but it really is only making the scary situation scarier! Anticipatory anxiety is useless worry.

3. Replace these thoughts with healthier, more balanced thoughts. Use positive self-talk to reassure yourself that you will be OK and that you can handle what comes your way (e.g., "I will be OK and I can handle what comes my way").

Exercises

Chapter 4 Exercise

Tips for Parents

1. When helping your child make the self-talk note cards, try to make them as specific to her fears as possible. The more personalized they are, the more effective they will be in helping your child manage her specific fears.

2. Self-talk statements are designed to help your child be able to effectively cope with the anxiety-provoking situation. In addition, self-talk often challenges their anxious automatic thoughts. Table 2 presents a list of sample self-talk statements organized by type of anxiety disorder, which you can use as a guide for helping your child make her note cards.

3. Try to get your child to practice relaxation at least three times this week (on three different days over the week). It would be ideal if your child practiced the calm breathing exercises three times, and did PMR once and relaxation imagery once this week. At least one of the three times should be on his own, without you present, as he ultimately needs to be able to use these skills on his own (e.g., when he is facing his fears). Encourage your child to use the calm breathing exercises anytime he feels or seems anxious or tense. If you have trouble getting your child to practice the relaxation or to do any of the exercises in this book, refer to Chapter 9, which discusses how to motivate your child to participate in the program.

Self-Talk Note Cards

Your exercise this week includes:

1. Making 8–10 self-talk note cards.
2. Making a list: "When the anxiety talks, it says . . . "
3. Keep practicing your relaxation (try to do it at least three times this week)

Exercises

Table 2
Self-Talk Note Cards Guide

Type of Anxiety Disorder	Positive Self-Talk Statement
Generalized Anxiety Disorder	"I can control my body. I can slow my breathing and calm my body."
	"I've worried in the past and it's been alright. This time is no different. It all will work out just fine."
	"It's just the anxiety talking. I am choosing not to listen to it."
	"I could cope with _____ if it happened. There is nothing I can't handle."
Separation Anxiety Disorder	"I am OK on my own. It will feel scary at first but then it will get better."
	"I am safe. I can always ask an adult at the party to help me if I need to."
	"I know it's hard to separate from _____(mom, dad), but I know I can do it. I know just how to soothe myself. I can _____(watch TV, bake with my babysitter, color, take a bath)."
Social Phobia	"How would someone who isn't anxious think or act in this situation?"
	"It is OK to look nervous in front of others. Everyone feels nervous from time to time."
	"How else can I explain what happened?"
	"Most people think favorable of others."
	"Can I think of times when my scary thoughts didn't come true?"
Specific Phobia	"Dogs are not dangerous. So many people wouldn't have them as pets if they were. My fears are irrational"
	"I am confident and relaxed and can touch the dog. Let me take a deep breath, then do it."
	"I must face my fears of snakes/spiders/dogs; I must do this to win and overcome my fears. I know I can do this."

Exercises

Type of Anxiety Disorder	Positive Self-Talk Statement
Obsessive-Compulsive Disorder	"It is just the OCD talking; if I listen and do what it says, it will win and I will lose. If I don't listen, I will win and the OCD will lose."
	"It's only a thought, it means nothing."
	"There is no proof that something bad will happen if I _____."
	"I must tolerate the anxious now in order to be less anxious in the long run. The anxiety may feel worse, but soon it will get better and go away."
	"Each time I _____(check, touch, count, etc), the OCD becomes stronger and wins."
	"The OCD thoughts are irrational. There is no point to _____(checking, touching, counting). I will be OK if I resist the urge to do it. The urge will pass and it will be fine."
Panic Disorder	"I don't need to be afraid of a panic attack. It feels uncomfortable but it is not dangerous."
	"I can handle feeling anxious."
	"Panic attacks are hard to handle, but I can do it. The panic will get better soon."
	"Nothing bad is happening to me. It just feels scary."
	"I can leave the situation for a few minutes, until I calm down, but then I must go back to the situation. I'm not going to let the panic interfere with what I am doing."

SELF-TALK NOTE CARDS

When making your note cards, you can use different colored index cards and you can add stickers to the note cards if you'd like. You can write them or have your mom or dad or write them—it's your choice. You will make five note cards like the ones below, and also make three to five of your own (you can make more if you'd like, but try to make at least three extra cards). The ones that you make on your own should be specific to you; they should be things that you can say to yourself that will help with your own specific worries and anxieties. Your mom or dad will help you with what to write.

Here are five note cards to make (make yours look just like these, with your own self-talk included):

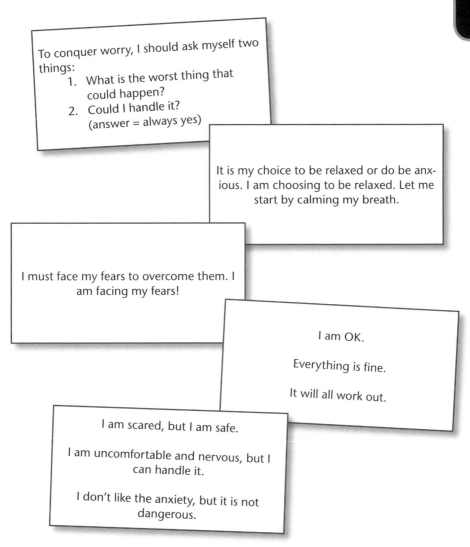

To conquer worry, I should ask myself two things:
1. What is the worst thing that could happen?
2. Could I handle it?
   (answer = always yes)

It is my choice to be relaxed or do be anxious. I am choosing to be relaxed. Let me start by calming my breath.

I must face my fears to overcome them. I am facing my fears!

I am OK.

Everything is fine.

It will all work out.

I am scared, but I am safe.

I am uncomfortable and nervous, but I can handle it.

I don't like the anxiety, but it is not dangerous.

IT'S THE ANXIETY TALKING

Remember James, the boy who was afraid of snakes? Well, when his anxiety was talking, it said things like:

"Snakes are scary and they will bite you."
"Don't go near the bushes, because a snake could be in there."
"That rustling sound was a snake."
"You can't go near snakes—they are the worst!"

James had to learn how to talk back to his anxiety, and he did this by knowing when his anxiety was talking to him and choosing not to listen to it! He told himself that the anxiety was wrong; then he told himself different things to help himself be able to face his fears. For example, he told himself that the rustling sound was most likely a squirrel or a bird. He reminded himself that most snakes don't bite humans. This is how he was able to face his fears and overcome his fear of snakes.

In the space below, write in some of the things that the anxiety says when you are feeling scared or anxious:

"When my anxiety talks, it says . . ."

_____

_____

_____

PRACTICE RELAXATION

Use the chart in the previous chapter to check off the days that you practiced and what type of relaxation you did.

CHAPTER

5

Changing Your Thoughts

In working toward overcoming her anxiety, Kimberly was taught that she had to change the way she thinks to change the way she feels. So, if she was to start feeling less anxious, she would need to start thinking differently. Kimberly did a lot of "What if . . . " thinking, which she learned was called "catastrophizing," a thinking mistake. She also made things seem worse, or a bigger deal, than they were, a thinking mistake called "magnifying," and had to do things her way or refused to do them at all, which was called "all-or-nothing" thinking. Kimberly began to catch herself making these thinking mistakes and challenged herself by trying to think differently and in a more flexible manner. Her parents helped her identify when she was making a thinking mistake, as they gently pointed it out to her when it happened.

I N this chapter, you and your child will learn about the different types of cognitive distortions or "thinking errors." You also will learn how to help your child change his anxious thoughts and beliefs (as a reminder, this chapter also is about the thoughts part of anxiety).

Let's start by understanding the connection between your thoughts and feelings. The way your child thinks about a situation impacts the way he will feel about it. For example, if he thinks that playing with your neighbor's dog is enjoyable and fun, he will feel excited. Yet, if he thinks that playing with your neighbor's dog is scary and frightening, he will feel anxious and scared.

The following examples are directly from your child's book:

Situation →	Thoughts →	Feelings
You are in front of your house and your neighbor is outside with her dog.	I really like dogs and can't wait to play with Sniffy. She's so cute!	Excited Happy Eager

Situation →	Thoughts →	Feelings
You are in front of your house and your neighbor is outside with her dog.	Dogs are so scary! I hope she doesn't come near me. If she comes toward me, I'll run inside!	Anxious Nervous Scared

Situation →	Thoughts →	Feelings
You are called on in class by the teacher to answer a question.	I feel comfortable being called on. I like to share my thoughts. Maybe the teacher will like my answer.	Relaxed Calm Enthusiastic

Situation →	Thoughts →	Feelings
You are called on in class by the teacher to answer a question.	I can't stand talking in front of the class. What if I say the wrong answer and everyone laughs and thinks I'm dumb?	Anxious Nervous Scared

Situation →	Thoughts →	Feelings
You have a big science test tomorrow and you have been studying for 3 days.	I am prepared and will probably do well because I have been studying a lot.	Calm Self-Assured Organized

Situation →	Thoughts →	Feelings
You have a big science test tomorrow and you have been studying for 3 days.	What if I fail? What if I forget everything I know? I will be in big trouble if I fail. The test is going to be impossible!	Anxious Nervous Scared

These examples illustrate that if something makes your child feel anxious, it has to do with the way he is thinking about it. Additionally, this means that your child can *change the way he thinks to change the way he feels*! This is an essential component to overcoming worry and anxiety. Remind him that he can do this, and that with practice, he will become proficient at it. When reviewing these concepts with your child, encourage him to consider that if the child in the above example were to change his thoughts and think like a nonanxious person, he would feel calm and relaxed. For instance, instead of thinking about failing the science exam and getting in big trouble, he could replace these thoughts with healthier ones like "I am prepared and I will probably do well because I have been studying a lot." Initially, your child may not believe these thoughts—they will feel unfamiliar and foreign; however, with practice and time, balanced, healthy thinking will become natural and automatic.

An important part of changing thoughts is to identify the specific cognitive errors that your child is making. This also will help your child identify patterns of her thinking. Thinking mistakes consistently result in negative feelings, such as anxiety and insecurity.

Types of Cognitive Distortions (Thinking Mistakes and Thinking Errors)

Everyone, including all children and adults, makes thinking mistakes or thinking errors. Thinking errors occur automatically and often exist outside of your child's awareness. Your child will learn that thinking errors are erroneous because they are inaccurate or irrational. In fact, most thinking errors made by your child are rooted in anxiety (and serve to reinforce anxiety). Tell your child that she should not feel bad about making thinking errors, and remind her that all children and adults make them. The following is a personal example that I share with your child in her book:

This past year I went to an island called Barbados and heard that there were really cool sea turtles in the ocean. The only thing was that you needed to take a speed boat to get to see them. So, I arranged for the hotel's motorboat to take us to see the sea turtles. Well, when the motorboat came up to the ocean shore to pick us up, I suddenly felt a rush of anxiety and fear and worry come over me. My heart started pounding, my stomach and knees felt weak, and I couldn't stop thinking about how scary it would feel going so fast on this boat—speeding along on the ocean. I worried that I would be so scared that I'd want to come back to shore, and that I wouldn't like it at all. I really felt too afraid to go. I told my husband Brian that I was so nervous that I wasn't sure I could go, and asked him if he thought it would be OK. Because Brian knows that I work with kids with anxiety and that I teach kids how to face their fears, he replied,

"Well, you need to face your fears," then jumped onto the boat! I decided to take his (really my) advice and got on the boat too. The next thing I know, we are speeding along on the ocean going very fast and the funny thing was, I had no anxiety at all. Not even the tiniest amount of fear. I probably couldn't have felt afraid if I tried. I was totally calm and relaxed and loved every minute of the boat ride. I loved the feeling of the ocean air against my face, the feeling of being on a boat, traveling on water, and looking at the beautiful island as we rode by. More than all of this, swimming with the sea turtles was one of the greatest times of my life! The sea turtles were huge and so interesting to watch as they swam in their ocean. It was a magical time and it would never have happened if I didn't face my fears.

It is clear that the thoughts I had about going on the boat and my physiological reaction of anxiety were not accurate predictors of my experience on the motorboat. My thoughts were actually thinking errors and the two specific ones I made were "probability overestimations" and "catastrophizing." This is a good example of how one thought can actually represent more than one thinking error.

Below is a list of 10 different thinking errors and examples of each (these also are listed in Appendix B: Thinking Errors Quick Reference Page). Note that most children with anxiety disorders tend to make several thinking errors on a consistent basis. When learning about the different types, try to consider which ones you have personally made and which ones you observe your child making:

1. **Catastrophizing:** Your child expects, even visualizes disaster. She notices or hears about a potential problem and thinks, "What if …" the worst thing happens. She also feels like she couldn't handle it if something bad did happen.

Example: Your child thinks, "What if I am scared on the motorboat and won't be able to calm down? What if we get stuck out in the middle of the ocean?"

Example: You are going out for dinner and your child asks, "Mommy, what if something bad happens to you?"

2. **All-or-Nothing:** Also known as black-and-white thinking, dichotomous thinking, and polarized thinking; when your child thinks in extremes—things are either perfect or a failure; there is no middle ground—it's either one extreme or another; thinking in an inflexible way.

   Example: Your child feels that if he doesn't get an A on the test, then he will fail the whole class and his report card will be ruined.

   Example: You planned on having pizza for dinner, but the pizza place closed so you brought home Chinese food instead. Your daughter is extremely upset about this and announces, "The whole day is ruined now! I'm not eating Chinese!"

3. **Filtering:** When your child focuses on the negative parts of a situation while ignoring the positive parts; she catches all of the bad parts and forgets about the good parts; she disqualifies the positive.

   Example: Your daughter goes to a birthday party and has a great time until the end when another kid says something mean to her. When you pick her up and ask how the party was, she tells you, "It was terrible. I had the worst time!"

   Example: Her report card arrives and she made all A's and B's but got one C in history. She is so upset and only focuses on her history grade; she ignores all of the other good grades that she earned and begins to cry about the C.

4. **Magnifying:** When your child makes something seem bigger and worse than it really is; he turns up the volume on anything bad, making it worse.

Example: You remind your son that he has a check-up at the doctor's tomorrow after school, and he begins to cry and tells you this is the worst news he has ever heard and he hates his life!

Example: A bug lands on your son's shirt and he screams at the top of his lungs and runs around trying to get it off.

5. **Shoulds:** Rules that your child has about the way things should be; when she uses the words "should," "must," and "ought to" to show how things should be.

   Example: Your daughter forgets to hand in a homework assignment. When she hands it in the next day, her teacher marks it down to a B because it is late. She becomes very upset with herself and thinks, "I shouldn't make mistakes like this. That was so stupid of me."

   Example: Your child has her friend Mary come over to play with her and she thinks that Mary should be willing to play whatever games she picks, because they are playing at her house. Your daughter picks out Monopoly but Mary doesn't want to play Monopoly and would rather play Clue, so your daughter becomes very upset with Mary because she believes that Mary should follow her rules. She then refuses to play anything other than Monopoly.

6. **Mind Reading:** When your child thinks she knows what others are thinking, particularly what they are thinking about her; usually she thinks that others are thinking negatively about her.

   Example: When she answers a question in class, your child thinks that other kids are thinking that she is stupid and doesn't know what she is talking about.

   Example: When her softball coach gives her a pointer, she believes that he thinks that she is the worst player on the team.

7. **Overgeneralization:** Your child takes a single incident and thinks that it always will be this way; something happens once and he thinks it will always happen in the same way.

    Example: He gets very nervous when giving a presentation on a book report. Afterward, he comments that he is not good at giving presentations and expects that he will always feels anxious when giving them.

    Example: You and your son go to an awards ceremony at his school but he doesn't get any awards. When leaving, he tells you that he is never going to an awards ceremony again because he won't get an award anyway, so what's the point?

8. **Personalization:** When your child takes something personally, she makes it about her when it has nothing to do with her. She takes responsibility when a negative outcome occurs, without considering other factors that may have contributed to it.

    Example: Your daughter walks by two girls in the lunchroom who are whispering and she thinks that they are whispering about her.

    Example: She didn't receive an invitation to her friend's birthday party so she thinks that her friend must be mad at her and doesn't want to be her friend anymore.

9. **Selective Attention:** Your child pays attention to things that confirm his beliefs about something; he ignores evidence that goes against what he believes about a particular situation.

    Example: He thinks that other kids don't like him and then he tells you about the time he was teased at recess and the time when his neighbor told him that she didn't want to play with him anymore. He doesn't think about the kids who do like him or about all of the fun times he had with his friends from the soccer team.

Example: His brother gets a new computer and he begins to think that you and his other parent don't get him anything, and how his computer is 2 years old. He doesn't think about how he recently got a new bed and that when he got his computer 2 years ago, his brother did not get one.

10. **Probability Overestimation:** Your child overestimates the likelihood that something bad will happen.

Example: Your daughter thinks that her presentation is going to be terrible and that she will be panicked the whole time.

Example: She is about to get on a motorboat and begins to think that she will be scared and anxious during the whole ride (does this sound familiar?).

It is common for certain anxiety disorders to be associated with certain thinking errors; however, any child can make any of the above thinking errors, regardless of his or her diagnosis. Table 3 specifies common thinking errors for each type of anxiety disorder.

In addition to the 10 cognitive distortions described above, there are several others that are specific to obsessive-compulsive disorder (OCD), and these are covered in the special section on OCD in Chapter 10.

Replacing Your Anxious Thoughts

After your child has identified her anxious thoughts, the next step is to change them. She can do this by replacing her thinking errors with more balanced, neutral thoughts. For example, instead of thinking that others are thinking bad things about her, she can think that most likely this is not the case. Instead of thinking about something bad happening to her mom or dad, she can think about

Table 3
Common Thinking Errors

Type of Anxiety Disorder	Common Thinking Errors
Generalized Anxiety Disorder	Catastrophizing, All-or-Nothing, Magnifying, Filtering
Separation Anxiety Disorder	Catastrophizing, Magnifying, Probability Overestimation
Social Phobia	Mind Reading, Personalization, Probability Overestimation, Shoulds, Selective Attention
Specific Phobia	Catastrophizing, Magnifying, Filtering, Probability Overestimation
Obsessive-Compulsive Disorder	All-or-Nothing, Catastrophizing, Shoulds, Probability Overestimation
Panic Disorder	Catastrophizing, Probability Overestimation

how her parents go out to dinner all the time and are always safe; she also can remind herself that going out to dinner is a safe activity. Instead of thinking that the whole day is ruined because her mom brought home Chinese food and not pizza, she can learn to think about the day more realistically and balance her disappointment about not having pizza with thoughts about how the rest of the day can be great.

To replace her thoughts, your child must "consider the facts" and ask herself, "What proof do I have that this thought is correct?" For example, what proof does she have that her mind reading is correct? How does she know that the other kids think she is stupid when she answers a question in class? How does she know how she will feel once she is speeding along the water on a motorboat? What proof does she have that her presentation will be a disaster? Even if she has given a not-so-fantastic presentation in the past, how does she know that this particular presentation will not go well? The *fact* is that she doesn't have any proof about what will happen in the future because it hasn't happened yet! Remind her that her worries are part of anticipatory anxiety; they are about future events that haven't occurred yet.

Chapter 5 Exercise

Tips for Parents

1. When helping your child complete this exercise, try to pick one of the less anxiety-provoking situations and one of the most anxiety-provoking situations on his ladder. If your child wants to use two of the harder situations, that is acceptable; however, using two of the easier situations will be a disadvantage because it will not provide the extra preparation for facing the more powerful fears.

2. Your child will need your help with identifying the thinking errors and with developing replacement thoughts. Reviewing all of the thinking errors with him will be beneficial and will help both of you to become more familiar with the different types. I also suggest that you highlight (with a highlighter) your child's most common thinking errors in his book. It also is recommended that you share some of your own personal examples of times that you have made thinking errors (if you have a hard time doing this, ask your child which thinking errors he or she thinks you most often make; you may be quite surprised to see how observant your child is when it comes to you!).

Identify and Replace Thinking Errors

Your exercise this week includes:

1. Listing two of your anxiety situations from your ladder and the anxious thoughts you have about these situations.

2. Labeling your thinking mistakes if there are any.

3. Changing your thoughts by creating "replacement thoughts," using the tool below. Remember: Replacement thoughts are balanced and neutral thoughts that do not cause anxiety. (*Hint*: You will know that you came up with a good replacement thought when the thought makes

you feel calmer and more prepared to cope with the scary situation).

Situation →	Thoughts →	Thinking Error(s)
	Replacement Thoughts:	

Situation →	Thoughts →	Thinking Error(s)
	Replacement Thoughts:	

Exercises

Situation →	Thoughts →	Thinking Error(s)

Replacement Thoughts:

Situation →	Thoughts →	Thinking Error(s)

Replacement Thoughts:

CHAPTER

6

Changing Your Behaviors

Facing Your Fears

To deal with her anxiety, Kimberly was skilled at avoiding certain situations, such as not being the first to walk into her house. She also regularly sought reassurance from her parents, would throw a tantrum when unexpected changes in the schedule occurred, and she scanned her environment at home for trouble, such as signs of a break-in or ways her dog could get loose. Kimberly and her parents identified these behaviors as anxious behaviors. She then systematically, by taking one step at a time, began to face her fears and gradually became more comfortable doing those things she avoided. When Kimberly asked for reassurance, her parents reminded her that they could not let the anxiety win by giving into it; if she asked if the dog was OK, her mom replied, "Kim, that's the anxiety talking. If I answer you, the anxiety will get stronger and win, and I can't do that as a member of your team." Kimberly sometimes got upset when her mom wouldn't answer, but deep down she knew her mom was right not to listen to the anxiety.

THIS chapter focuses on preparing your child to face her fears. By now, you and your child have learned about the body and thoughts parts of anxiety; this chapter is on the third part: behavior.

Chapter 5 illustrated how thoughts influence feelings; it also is true that feelings influence behavior. Therefore, if your child *feels* afraid of something, she will probably try to avoid it. Children demonstrate other nervous behaviors when they are anxious, including but not limited to the following:

- reassurance seeking (asking you or another adult for validation or affirmation that a situation is safe and that they are OK);
- clinging (staying near you or another adult);
- crying;
- picking (nails, hair, feet, lips, or any other part of one's body);
- fidgeting;
- freezing;
- having a tantrum or meltdown;
- scanning their environment (looking around for signs that make them feel more relaxed); and
- rituals (repetitive behaviors typically done to reduce anxiety).

As previously explained, avoidance behavior reinforces anxiety about the situation and in general. To overcome your child's anxiety, you and your child cannot engage in avoidance behavior anymore. I say "you" because most caring parents enable their child to avoid her fearful situations. This is referred to as *accommodation;* you are accommodating her fears to prevent her from having a negative emotional experience. As mentioned in Chapter 2, accommodating your child's anxiety and providing reassurance are common acts of loving, caring parents; however, this behavior is damaging to your child as it prevents her from facing of her fears and confirms for her that the situation she dreads is worth fearing.

Remind your child of the "you against the fear" mindset and encourage her to take a positive attitude. Tell her that she can do this and that she will win! In review, your child will begin at the bottom of her ladder (hierarchy) and will gradually move up, going from least to most anxiety-provoking. Occasionally, children do not accurately rank their fears or an opportunity to do one of the steps presents itself (i.e., they get invited to a sleepover and this is one of their steps), and the two of you will decide to deviate from the order and structure of the ladder. This is perfectly fine, as long as you generally follow with the sequence and your child is willing to make this deviation. The main idea is that you do not want your child to face a high-anxiety fear when she is not ready and then have a bad experience in which she is terrified, as this will likely strengthen the anxiety.

Each step on the ladder is called an *exposure*, because your child is being exposed to the anxiety-provoking situation. It is imperative that your child not be forced to do the exposures. Although you can provide encouragement, and maybe even push a little, if you force her to do an exposure, her anxiety may be unintentionally strengthened. If getting your child to cooperate with facing her fears is challenging, refer to Chapter 9, which focuses on motivating your child. If your child is still not cooperative, it may be that the first step is too difficult for her to start with and you may need to help her come up with an easier step, or break the step down into much smaller parts. In fact, breaking the steps into smaller parts or making them "time-limited" (start with doing it for 1 minute) is a good idea for many children, as it makes the task more manageable. Usually, once children begin to face their fears and have success in doing so, it becomes much easier to get them to face the rest of their fears on the ladder.

Also, I have shared the following good news with your child in his book:

Once you are done facing all of your fears, there will be a celebration in your honor. You and your parent(s) are going to have a little party to celebrate you and all of your hard work. You may even get an award or a special treat! You might decide to invite a sibling if you have one or a best friend or grandparent to celebrate you with you and your parent.

Remind your child that he is prepared to handle facing his fears and the feelings of anxiety that may arise during the process. He has tools and strategies for coping and also has your support. As he faces his fears, make sure to give a lot of praise and positively reinforce his effort and successes. In addition, encourage him to praise and compliment his success. You and your child together should place the stickers on his hierarchy for each step that he has completed. It is recommended that you point to where he should put the sticker, but he should be the one to actually place it on the ladder.

The exercise this week is designed to help your child review the strategies he has learned to help manage or cope with his anxiety. It is normal for him to experience anxiety as he begins to face his fears. Most children will find that after some initial anxiety, their anxiety significantly decreases as they continue to stick with the exposures. Ultimately, he will experience no anxiety as he will become desensitized and habituated. I explained to your child in his book that the children I work with always feel great after they face their fears and often report how surprised they were to find that the exposures were not as terrifying as they had expected. This realization also will help motivate your child to continue to face his more challenging fears listed at the top part of his ladder.

You and your child will create a *plan for coping* to prepare him for the exposures. You may need to review this plan several times with him, especially in the beginning; however, if it becomes so repetitive that it resembles reassurance seeking, I recommend that you ask *him* to tell *you* the plan. A plan for coping with the exposures will increase his sense of preparation.

Plan for Coping

A plan for coping will consistently include using the strategies or tools in your child's toolbox that will help him deal with his anxiety. The tools your child has learned in the previous chapters include:

- calm breathing;
- progressive muscle relaxation;
- relaxing imagery;
- conquer worry (understanding when worry is useless; asking yourself two things; using the big picture perspective; scheduling worry time);
- positive self-talk;
- talking back to the anxiety;
- dealing with anticipatory anxiety (label, remind, and replace);
- self-talk note cards (including "you must face your fears to overcome them"); and
- changing your thoughts (identifying and replacing thinking errors).

Most likely, your child won't use *every* tool in *his* toolbox, just his favorites and most effective ones. Plus, he will likely use different tools for different situations. For example, James (the boy who had a snake phobia) used calm breathing as he looked at pictures of snakes in a book, but he used conquer worry and positive self-talk tools when he stood near a live snake.

When doing the exposures, you may find that your child becomes so anxious and panicked that he is unable to effectively use the strategies like conquering worry and changing his thoughts. If this happens, encourage him to use distraction techniques in addition to calm breathing to calm down enough to be able to conquer worries and change his thoughts. Examples of distraction techniques include:

▸ Using the ABCs to calm down: Your child can go through the alphabet and try to come up with a different girl's name for each letter (e.g., Amy, Bonnie, Camryn, Denise, Emily, Frances). Or, she could do this for boy's names, cities, countries, places, types of foods, or types of jobs (e.g., artist, baker, chemist, dentist, environmentalist, firefighter). This will help distract her from the anxiety-provoking situation.

▸ Focusing: Your child can focus on something that she can see (e.g., a tree, book, sneakers) and try to think of five or more different parts of it or ways to describe it (e.g., What color is it? What shape is it? What does it smell like? What does it sound like? What does it feel like? What could you use it for?).

▸ Pick a color and think of five things that come in that color.

▸ Singing: Your child could sing a song to herself or make up a rhyme in her head.

▸ Counting: Your child could count backward from 100 by 7 (e.g., 100, 93, 86, 79, . . .) or any other number.

Another part of making a plan for coping during exposures is to decide if your child wants to break down the exposure into even smaller steps, as mentioned above. For instance, when James did his first exposure (talking about snakes) he began by talking about snakes for 1 minute, then did it again the next day for 5 minutes, then did it again on the third day for 10 minutes.

When facing your fears, review what your plan will involve with your child: Think about which tools he will use and which distraction technique he will rely on if using the tools becomes difficult to accomplish.

When it comes time for your child to do an exposure, he should rate his anxiety on a scale from 0–10. He can rate his anxiety level on a "FEAR-mometer" scale.

0 = no fear at all/completely relaxed like in a deep sleep

5 = nervous and scared but not too terrible

10 = extremely afraid, totally anxious, and maybe panicked

It is essential that when your child is doing the exposures, that *you* remain completely calm. If he detects that you are anxious, he may feel that there is good reason to feel anxious and have trouble calming down. Be calm and be very encouraging; Display confidence in your child and praise him for each step taken toward facing his fears.

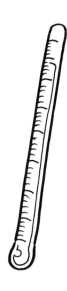

Chapter 6 Exercise

Tips for Parents

1. When your child is writing the tools in his toolbox, make sure that he has included most of the tools listed on page 91. When noting his fear level, you can do this verbally, "On a scale from 0–10, where was your anxiety?" Alternatively, you and your child can draw a picture of the FEAR-mometer and he can write in the exposure at the point on the ladder that represents his anxiety level. It also is important for your child to note the changes in his anxiety level (from 0–10) after he stays present in an exposure (e.g., he may start out with an "8" but after 5 minutes he may be down to a "4") and as he continues to do the same exposure on different occasions (e.g., the first time James looked at pictures of snakes he rated his fear at a "6" but by the fourth time, he rated it as a "1 or 2" because he became used to looking at pictures of snakes).

2. After each exposure, remind your child of his change in anxiety level (e.g., "You did a great job, and your anxiety went down from an 8 to a 4"). The goal is for your child to do each exposure repeatedly—not just once or twice. Ultimately, we want the exposure to cause your child no anxiety, and this will be accomplished with practice, repetition, and prolonged exposure.

3. Generally, your child will earn two stars for each exposure (each placed on one side of the ladder for that particular step). The first star will be earned after your child does the exposure for the first time. The second star will be given once your child has practiced the exposure several times and the situation no longer evokes a sense of anxiety. The second star symbolizes that your child has overcome that particular fear or anxiety.

Facing Your Fears

Your exercise this week includes:

1. Drawing a picture of a toolbox and writing the different "tools" you can use to control your anxiety in your toolbox. (Remember, the tools are the different strategies you can use to manage your anxiety; they are all listed earlier in this chapter.)

2. Taking the first step of your ladder (do your first exposure).

   ▶ Remember to put stickers on your ladder after you have practiced your first step several times!

   ▶ Remember to note what your anxiety level was on the FEAR-mometer.

Make your picture of the toolbox look something like this one:

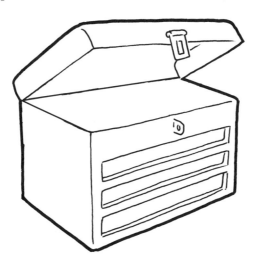

CHAPTER

7

Keep Facing Your Fears

After taking the first step on her ladder—only checking on her dog twice a day—Kimberly was ready to take the next step. Although it was a challenge for her to hold back her urge to check, she relied on her coping plan to help her deal with the exposure. Kimberly used calm breathing, positive self-talk, and distraction to cope with her feelings of anxiety. The longer she went without checking, the easier it was to not check. Kimberly then took her next step on the ladder: doing homework while staying calm. She developed a system of writing down her assignments in checklist form and estimating how long each one would take. She checked off the completed assignments as she went along, reassuring herself that she could handle it and would only focus on the one task at hand. With practice, Kimberly learned to be calm when doing her daily homework. Her parents were very supportive and cheered her on, complimenting her for earning stars on her ladder!

THIS chapter also is on the behavior part of anxiety. If you are reading this chapter, it most likely means that your child has faced his or her first fear, so let me officially congratulate you for being so effective in helping your child overcome his anxiety! Taking the first step is a big step for your child, and you should feel very proud of him for getting this far. You also should feel proud of yourself for helping your child get here.

As you can probably predict, the goal at this point is for your child to continue to take the rest of the steps on the ladder one at a time, and the exercise at the end of this chapter is focused on preparing your child to accomplish this. (Remember that Chapter 9 provides guidance on how to motivate your child to complete this program, including how to help her face her fears.) Once all of the steps are taken on the ladder, your child can go on to Chapter 8 (which is the last chapter in his book) and celebrate his success!

Remind your child that while facing his fears is difficult to do, he will feel much better as a result, and also will gain freedom from his anxiety! Soon his anxiety will not dictate how he will feel or think or act, nor will it dictate how *you* will act. In addition, by facing his fears, your child will feel much better about himself and his self-confidence will strengthen and improve.

It is essential that you encourage your child to feel proud of herself, as this is an indication of healthy self-esteem. Self-esteem develops when children gain mastery in a certain area, including facing their fears. It is important that parents facilitate opportunities for their child to gain mastery, and when a child has achieved mastery, that parents make her aware that this has occurred. Take a moment to think about areas in which your child exhibits strong ability and make a commitment to help him use this ability as much as possible. When he engages in such mastery, point it out to him at the appropriate time. For example, comments such as, "Your excellent math skills really helped you do well on the test. I can tell from your teacher's comments that she was really impressed," "You are a true musician. Your piano playing was fantastic—did you hear everyone clapping after your performance? You should be very proud of yourself," and "You are such an excellent chef! I've never tasted cookies so good. Will you make these again for our party next week?" can help your child recognize his strengths. Also, if you feel that your child does not seem to naturally have mastery in any particular area, it is equally important for you to cultivate such opportunities (e.g., encourage your child to make a lemonade stand or get him involved in some charity work, such as for the Humane Society; this will be rewarding in many ways). Finally, listening to your child and validating her opinions, preferences, and feelings also is quite important. It is crucial not to judge your child for her feelings; she should learn from you that feelings are not good or bad or right or wrong; rather, feelings just are what they are, and feelings must be respected. A parent can judge his child's behavior as good or bad, but parents must tread carefully: Children should not get the message that *they* are bad, rather, it should be made clear that it was their *behavior* that was inappropriate. Finally, it is recommended that you model the skill of "forgiving and moving on," allowing opportunities for a fresh start.

A parent's role in the development of his child's self-esteem is profound. Self-esteem is one of the strongest predictors of success and happiness in adulthood, and I would argue it is far more important than the type of school or college your child will attend. Praising your child is necessary, although overpraise (too much praise and praise for unimportant events) may be counterproductive as it may cause children to question the authenticity of deserving praise.

Keeping in mind that anxiety breeds self-doubt, which may weaken or threaten self-esteem, overcoming anxiety can be an incredibly powerful boost to your child's confidence in himself. I strongly encourage you to incorporate this aspect into your child's process of overcoming his anxieties and fears. Your child will learn the following about self-esteem:

Self-esteem refers to how you feel about yourself and it can either be good (healthy) or bad (unhealthy). Kids with good self-esteem feel proud of themselves and their accomplishments and they know what they are good at doing. Also, they don't forget how good they are when things don't work out well for them. For example, they don't beat themselves up for their mistakes or when they don't do as well as they would like to do. And, when others say mean things about them, like some kids do, they don't believe it—they don't forget that they are a good, special person. Like anxiety, which has three parts, self-esteem also has three parts:

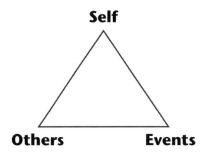

- ▸ The "Self" part, which is the most important of the three parts, means that you know and own your strengths; you know what is wonderful and special about you and you remember these qualities even on bad days. You know what you are good at doing, whether it's playing an instrument, dancing, or being a great athlete or an excellent speller.
- ▸ The "Others" part means that other people can help you feel good about yourself; your parents, friends, and teachers can compliment you or show they care about you and this will make you feel good about yourself. They can support you and help you know your positive strengths and areas to work on and improve upon. For example, your teacher can help you understand what your strengths are and also ways to become even better at your schoolwork.
- ▸ The "Events" part means that certain things can happen to you or certain things that you do can help you feel great about yourself; facing your fears counts as one of

these events. Other examples are when you study hard for a test and earn an A or when you score a goal for your team, or when you earn a green belt in karate.

When facing her fears, it is very important that your child cheer herself on and encourage herself to do the very thing she is afraid of. If she doubts her ability to do it, remind her that anxiety breeds self-doubt, and self-doubt breeds more self-doubt. The only antidote for self-doubt is proving to herself that she can do it by facing her fears. Boost her with encouraging comments: "I know you can do this," "You will succeed," "You will earn your stickers," "Remember that you can handle this, and it might not be as bad as you think it will be," and "I believe in you, and you will win!" Once your child succeeds, help her recognize and appreciate her success.

When facing her fears, try to encourage your child to stay mostly in the order of her ladder. Sometimes children may skip around and this is perfectly fine, as long as your child feels ready for it. However, it's usually not a good idea to do the steps at the top until you've at least done some of the ones in the bottom and middle. Most children find that by sticking close to the order of the steps, the exposures are more manageable. Sometimes children realize that they did not order their steps correctly, or they may feel differently about the situations after reading the first six chapters of their book; in either of these cases, skipping around may be appropriate. In addition, if an opportunity to do one of her steps arises (e.g., she is invited to a sleepover or a birthday party, or it's time to register for summer camp), your child might want to take advantage of the chance to take these steps, even if it requires her to go out of order on her ladder. Again, the primary consideration is that your child feels reasonably ready to take these steps. Feeling ready, of course, does not mean that she feels no anxiety about doing it, but instead means that she is willing to try, and perhaps can imagine being able to do it. For the majority of children, once they begin the process of taking the steps and facing their fears, they will have an easier time doing the rest of the steps. Motivating your child in the beginning will be your biggest challenge.

This also is the appropriate time to work with your child on getting rid of his nervous behaviors, as discussed in Chapter 6. Your child most likely has been doing these nervous behaviors for quite some time and thus, you have been used to dealing with them and responding to them for quite some time. The behaviors have been reinforcing for your child, as they have likely provided some relief to his anxiety. For example, clinging to you or getting reassurance that it will all be OK has made your child (temporarily) feel more safe and secure but these behaviors work to strengthen your child's overall anxiety. The best approach to helping your child stop these behaviors is a gradual one, similar to the idea of taking one step at a time on the ladder. Once your child has accomplished three or four steps, it is a good time to introduce the goal of gradually stopping the nervous behaviors. As the parent, you likely will be the one to initiate this process, and your child will benefit from your emotional support as she begins to end this unhealthy pattern of coping. Although you can reassure your child that he is capable of stopping and replacing these nervous behaviors, you cannot continue to reassure him in response to his anxiety-driven requests.

The first step in helping your child get rid of these behaviors is to point out when they are happening: Help your child become aware of when she is engaging in these behaviors. Label the behaviors as part of the anxiety. In your child's book, he will learn that you will eventually stop giving him the reassurance he seeks and that you are not doing this to upset or punish him. Remind him that providing the reassurance only serves to validate and strengthen the anxiety. Instead, as the parent, you will encourage your child to use his self-talk and relaxation skills to *help himself* feel better.

One option to help modify these nervous behaviors is to use a calendar to track each day that your child does not exhibit the nervous behaviors. For example, before bed, Billy repeatedly asked his mom if he could stay home from school the next day; sometimes she would give in and let him. After coming to therapy, Billy's mom learned that letting him stay home from school was actually making his anxiety worse. His mother then learned to change the way she responded to Billy, and instead she would say, "You sound nervous about going to school, but you have to go. What can you do to calm down, and how can I make it better for you?" At first, Billy didn't like this response from his mother, but after a while he got used to it and began to feel alright. They charted his progress on a calendar: Every night that Billy did not ask his mom if he could stay home from school, he earned a check on his calendar. Gradually, he learned that everything turned out fine, even though his mother did not allow him to stay home from school. Additionally, Billy recognized that he felt more confident because he was able to handle his anxiety and worries on his own. He also found school less stressful because he began attending regularly and was able to stay on top of his schoolwork.

Like Billy, your child can get rid of his nervous behaviors and feel better about himself. I recommend that you make a list of which nervous behaviors you observe your child doing, and then help your child gradually reduce the frequency and intensity of each behavior.

Exercises

Chapter 7 Exercise

Tips for Parents

1. In reference to the rest of the steps on the ladder, it will be extremely beneficial if you and your child can generate additional "replacement thoughts" for as many of the remaining anxiety-provoking situations on the ladder. Try to identify the thinking errors that your child is using that maintain his fear of the situation, then come up with a new, more balanced thought. It is not necessary to do this for each and every step on the ladder; however, at minimum, it should be done for the hardest steps and the ones that your child is most resistant to facing. Remind you child that we can change the way we think to change the way we feel. The exercise at the end of this chapter includes a chart that you and your child can use to develop replacement thoughts for the different anxiety-provoking situations.

2. You and your child should look at his toolbox before the exposures as a review of what he can do to cope with the anxiety that may arise in the process.

3. If your child struggles to complete a certain step, you may want to break the step down into even smaller steps to make it more manageable. For example, if your child has separation anxiety and one of his steps is to go to the bathroom alone, you may want to start with having him go into the bathroom alone and then you can come in halfway through. Then the next time, you would come in when you hear the toilet flush. In other words, you are helping him create smaller goals to work toward completing the step. It is best to define progress as any movement, no matter how gradual, toward the goal. Behavior change usually happens in small steps. Another example would be if your child has social anxiety and one of her steps includes going

to a birthday party. You can break this down into smaller steps, starting with going to a party for 30 minutes, then going to another party for 1 hour, and finally going for the full duration. Alternatively, you can make the exposure more manageable by giving her the option of calling you to come to the party (not to pick her up, but to be there as a support) if it is too challenging for her (in this case, you may drop your child off then go to a café close to the party location). These types of accommodations are appropriate to use during the exposure phase, and there is a time-limited nature to offering these accommodations; most importantly, they are offered solely for the purpose of helping your child complete the steps, which are a necessary part of the treatment process.

4. It is normal for children to feel anxious and scared the first couple of times they do a step on their ladder, but you can assure them that it will get easier with practice. This type of assurance is appropriate because it is done in support of the exposure process. In contrast, many children find that they are not anxious or scared at all when they take one of their steps, and when this happens, it is advantageous to help them understand that the anxiety they felt before they practiced was nothing more than anticipatory anxiety. This anxious feeling was not a good predictor of the actual experience.

5. One final note about completing the rest of the steps on your ladder: The goal is for your child to repeat each step on his ladder multiple times. Children don't just do a step once or twice and then forget about it. Instead, they continue to do it over and over until it no longer makes them feel anxious or scared, with the goal of the behavior becoming integrated into their normal repertoire of behaviors. This also will help to expand your child's comfort zone. So, once your child does something on her ladder, she will

Exercises

continue to do it repeatedly and then it will become something that she is able to do comfortably. Finally, it is best if the exposures are prolonged; the longer she stays in the situation, the better.

Good luck with helping your child on the rest of the steps!

Finish Your Ladder

1. Remember to go at your own pace, but try to do 1–2 steps each week.
2. Don't forget to:
   - put stickers on your ladder next to the step after you've taken it, and
   - note what your anxiety level was on the FEAR-mometer.
3. Change the way you think to change the way you feel! Use steps from your ladder for the situation and write down the automatic thought or worry you have about facing that fear. Then, figure out which thinking error you might have used, and come up with a new, more balanced and accurate thought for your replacement thought. Your parents can help you come up with these new thoughts. When you take each step, try to remind yourself of the replacement thought you came up with for that situation. Good luck!

Exercises

Situation →	Thoughts →	Thinking Error(s)

Replacement Thoughts:

Situation →	Thoughts →	Thinking Error(s)

Replacement Thoughts:

Situation →	Thoughts →	Thinking Error(s)

Replacement Thoughts:

Situation →	Thoughts →	Thinking Error(s)

Replacement Thoughts:

CHAPTER

8

Lessons Learned

Celebrate Yourself

With dedication and her parents' support, Kimberly successfully faced all of her fears. She practiced having unexpected changes in the schedule, and when it came time for her next dentist appointment, Kimberly's mother deliberately did not tell her until she picked her up from school. Unlike the last time, Kimberly was able to handle it and she went to the appointment without preparation. She knew that by doing so, she was not letting anxiety rule her life. Kimberly also got used to being the first one to walk into the house, and her heartbeat no longer increased as she did so. She stopped checking on her dog, and homework was a much more pleasant experience. Kimberly and her parents celebrated her great achievement: She completed her ladder and gained freedom from anxiety. There were some bumps in the road along the way, but Kimberly persevered, and overcame her fears. Kimberly and her parents celebrated with a special dinner at her favorite pizza place in her honor. At dinner, her parents shared how proud they were of all of her hard work and great success!

WELCOME to the last chapter of your child's book. Making it here is a tremendous accomplishment and both you and your child deserve a huge "Congratulations!"

In honor of completing this program, you will throw a little party (or the like) to celebrate all of your child's hard work and success, and you will present him with the official Certificate of Achievement (located on p. 82 in your child's book). Your child has the option of decorating the certificate, but I recommend that you fill in the lines with your child's name, date, and sign it. For the celebration, you and your child can invite other family members like siblings and grandparents, or you can keep it to just the two (or three if his other parent is included) of you. Some children like to have a party at home or prefer to do something else as their celebration, like going to a favorite place or favorite restaurant or doing a special activity. The celebration can be whatever you and your child decide upon; the only requirement is that it is in your child's honor. The party/celebration is a great time to further compliment your child for his excellent participation in this program and help him become aware of the mastery he has gained in the process.

Before the celebration, there are two final areas to address:

1. What lessons did you and your child learn?
2. How can your child handle anxiety and worries if they come up again in the future?

Lessons Learned

Let's review what your child did to get to the point of facing his fears and overcoming his anxiety.

First, your child learned about the three parts of anxiety: body, thoughts, and behavior. After creating his team and team goals and making the ladder, he learned how to work on each of the three parts in order to overcome his anxiety. To address the physiological component of anxiety, your child learned and practiced:

1. calm breathing,
2. progressive muscle relaxation, and
3. relaxing imagery.

To help with his anxious thoughts, he learned:
1. how to master his worries;
2. how to use self-talk;
3. about the situation-thought-feeling connection (how you think will affect how you feel, so changing your thoughts can change the way you feel); and
4. about thinking errors and how to change them to healthy replacement thoughts.

Finally, to help with the behavioral component, your child learned how to face her fears, one by one, and she did it by completing the steps on her ladder. She also learned how to get rid of other anxious behaviors and practiced eliminating those as well. Most importantly, your child learned that changing the way she thinks not only changed the way she feels, but it also changed the way she behaved!

By facing his fears, your child learned that he could beat anxiety and overcome it. Children who successfully face their fears also tend to realize that their fears were not as terrible as they anticipated that they would be. Thus, when they were in the different anxiety-provoking situations, they discovered that it was not that bad after all. They stayed with the situation and did not engage in avoidance behavior, and then became used to it; they were able to tolerate feared situations without being afraid.

Your child also learned that when presented with a challenge or obstacle, she can face it and become stronger as a result. Most children experience an improvement in their self-confidence from facing their fears and overcoming anxiety. In this way, they took back the control in their life and became free from the constraints of anxiety-avoidance behavior.

As a parent, you learned not to reinforce your child's fears by accommodating the anxiety. You learned that accommodating the anxiety made it worse, and you challenged your child (and yourself) by not giving in and by remaining firm. In this way, you were an instrumental part of your child's treatment plan. Without your willpower and insights, your child would not have been able to successfully overcome his anxiety.

Handling Worry and Anxiety in the Future (Relapse Prevention)

The majority of children who successfully learn the skills related to understanding and overcoming their anxiety and face their fears do not return to the state of anxiety that they were in at the onset of treatment. In other words, most children do not return to being as anxious as they were when they started the program. However, some children do have relapses (most of the time, these relapses are relatively small and easily worked through). The best part is, if this happens, you and your child know exactly what to do! Your child can handle any future anxiety in the same manner as she did throughout this program. You and your child now have the skills to deal with any anxiety. These skills are yours and can be used at any point in the future.

The following is an example given in your child's book:

James successfully overcame his fear of snakes by completing this program. More than a year went by without thinking about or worrying about snakes when James went to a birthday party and there was a snake trainer there to put on a show (can you believe it?). Because he had not thought about snakes for so long, when he first saw the huge snake around the neck of the trainer, James suddenly felt a rush of fear. For a moment, he forgot that he was no longer scared of snakes! Then he realized that he knew what to do: He knew that he needed to stay at the party, and actually sat closer to the snake trainer to make it more like he was facing his fears. He also took a few deep breaths and remembered that he could handle this. He reminded himself that he would be OK and that he's done this before so he can do it now. After about 5 minutes, James felt back to normal again. He was calm and felt no fear. James was reminded that whenever he felt anxious, he just needed to use the tools in his toolbox and face his fears. Like James, you may have some anxiety and worry from time to time. Just do what you have throughout this program, and you'll be fine. Keep this book someplace safe and come back to it whenever you need to. I know that everything will work out for you, and I wish you all the best in your future.

The key to preventing relapse is to encourage your child to face any fears that may arise in the future. As soon as you observe any avoidance behavior, try to nip it in the bud by having your child face his fears. Some children have returned for tune-up appointments and some present with a few (and often new) anxieties or fears. For these children, I often will make another "mini-ladder," with two to four steps on it to address the anxiety-provoking situations, and will have them review their self-talk note cards and other exercises (at the end of each chapter). Because they have successfully completed the treatment and have overcome their past fears, this process is generally very smooth and only takes a short time.

Keep in mind that not all things that your child doesn't want to do is a fear; sometimes it is simply a preference. For example, a girl with social anxiety may prefer to only invite one friend over at a time. Although this could be interpreted as anxiety (e.g., she is afraid to have more than one friend over at a time), it could likely be that she just prefers to invite only one friend rather than inviting more friends over at the same time. Asking your child for clarification, "Is this something that makes you feel uncomfortable or nervous, or this is something you like better?" and scanning for visible signs of anxiety are the best ways to assess the situation. Also, look for signs of anxiety, such as what the child says about the event (e.g., is he describing worries or concerns about it?) or if he exhibits other nervous behaviors.

Chapter 8 Exercise

Tips for Parents

1. The party and receiving the Certificate of Achievement is an important part of your child's participation in the program. The concept of rewarding oneself, celebrating one's achievements, and feeling positive about accomplishing hard work is an important component for healthy self-esteem development. This is your chance to model this for your child and help your child celebrate herself!

2. The details of the party will be discussed by you and your child. It does not have to involve spending a lot of money; rather, the spirit of the celebration is what counts.

3. Some parents choose to frame their child's certificate after it is completed and/or decorated.

Celebrate Yourself With a Party and Earn Your Official Certificate of Achievement!

1. Talk to your mom or dad about the party and who should come to it. Some kids have the party with just their moms or dads, and others invite their siblings, pets, or friends. There is no right or wrong way to do it—the only rule is that you have fun and celebrate all of your hard work and success!

2. For the Certificate of Achievement, you and your parent can complete the form and you can decorate it anyway you like! Have a great party—you deserve it!

CHAPTER

9

Motivating
Your Child

OST parents will benefit from reading this chapter early on in the course of this program. This chapter offers several different approaches to help motivate your child to read the book, do the exercises, and face her fears. The goal is to be able to complete the program as a self-help resource; however, if after implementing the techniques described in this chapter you are unable to get your child engaged in the process, I recommend that you seek professional help. The Resources for Parents section at the end provides links to finding an appropriate therapist in your area. It is important that you do not force your child to read the book and/or complete the program.

The ideal age range for this companion series is 7–14. Some of the motivational techniques described in this chapter will be more appropriate for younger children while others will be more appropriate for early teens. Finally, some children will get stuck on not wanting to read the book and others will show resistance toward doing the exposures. Therefore, this chapter is divided into five sections:

1. general principles of reinforcement,
2. motivational strategies for younger children not willing to read the chapters,
3. motivational strategies for younger children not willing to do the exposures,
4. motivational strategies for early teens not willing to read the chapters, and
5. motivational strategies for early teens not willing to do the exposures.

General Principles of Reinforcement

First, let me clarify that I do not believe that the treatment of childhood anxiety disorders should incorporate discipline strategies—this is not a behavioral problem in the classic sense. Rather, childhood anxiety disorders describe a mental condition that often involves a great deal of pain and discomfort. Being punished for not being able to face one's fears only serves to exacerbate this pain and discomfort. Although most children with anxiety disorders have symptoms that are not visible (e.g., internal thoughts, self-talk, self-doubt), some children's anxiety manifests as tantrums and meltdowns. However, these are unlike the tantrums and meltdowns that we often see in children who cannot get their way, as the behavior is rooted in a very strong drive to avoid anxiety-provoking situations. It is essential to understand the causes of a child's disruptive behavior.

The sections below will provide guidance on how to deal with a child's unwillingness to read the chapters and/or do the exposures. Some children with anxiety disorders also are oppositional in general (and this oppositionality typically is observed in circumstances when the child is *not* anxious or *not* in an anxiety-provoking situation), and these children may require discipline strategies to address the oppositionality in order to help them comply with the program. However, once they comply with the program they may want to avoid the exposures, and disciplining this anxious behavior is *not* appropriate.

In general, reinforcement is used to increase the occurrence of a behavior and the behavior we are targeting is participation in this program. Positive reinforcement describes the act of rewarding a child with something desirable once he has done a good job. For example, if your child washes your car and you give your child $5, he is more likely to wash your car again because he enjoyed earning the money. Negative reinforcement describes the act of removing something undesirable once he has done a good job. For example, if your child washes your car and as a result does not have to do any other chores like the laundry or cleaning his room, he is more likely to wash your car again because he avoided doing something that he found unpleasant. Both positive and negative reinforcement are used in this program. The use of positive reinforcement, in particular, will help your child be cooperative with this program.

Examples of positive reinforcement include earning rewards for reading chapters and completing the exposures, giving your child praise for his cooperation and hard work, and, most importantly, being able to do activities he previously avoided because he is no longer afraid to do them! Earning rewards is a great bonus for many children. Although some children will not seek rewards and will be willing to do it simply because they are asked to (perfectionistic children may be more likely to fall into this category), many will benefit greatly from a reward plan. I recommend that rewards be mostly activity-based rather than monetarily-based; however, I see little wrong with having some of the latter. Negative reinforcement has an important role as well—doing the exposures naturally results in the removal of unpleasant anxiety, and therefore your child will be more motivated to do additional exposures.

Motivational Strategies for Younger Children Not Willing to Read the Chapters

Prior to implementing any of the strategies below, I recommend that you attempt to understand your child's resistance to beginning the program. There are many potential and understandable explanations for his unwillingness to start. For instance, your child may simply be afraid of the idea of change (many anxious children resist change and transitions in general), or he may not be willing to recognize the impairment that results from having the anxiety, or he may not like the idea of having to actually do the work of dealing with the anxiety (think of how many adults resist going to therapy because the thought of addressing their problems seems too daunting!). Try to validate your child's feelings and concerns, then boost him up with encouragement and rational statements such as, "I know the idea of doing this seems like a lot—even overwhelming to you—but your worries (or fears or anxiety) are a problem and we need to work together to fix them," "I'm going to do my part, too. See, I have my own book that I'll be reading while you read yours," and "We're going to take one chapter at a time, and we can come up with a reward system to help you feel more excited about it."

Draw a table similar to that in Table 4.

Show your child the table and explain that she will earn a check for each chapter she reads and for each exercise she completes. Explain that the number of checks earned will equal a privilege or reward of some kind, then generate a "Reward List" (see p. 121). Once your child gets to Chapters 7 and 8, she will begin earning stars on her ladder so she will have the opportunity to earn additional points (stars/checks) for rewards.

Create a Rewards List similar to the one on the next page. Your child should participate in selecting the rewards and creation of the list, although it's your job to ensure that the rewards are appropriate for the number of stars/points.

Table 4
Reward Chart

	Read Chapter	Did Exercise
Chapter 1		
Chapter 2		
Chapter 3		
Chapter 4		
Chapter 5		
Chapter 6		
Chapter 7		
Chapter 8		

James's Reward List

Number of Stars (or Points)	Reward
2	Pick a toy from the toy basket
3	30 minutes computer time
4	Watch a movie with mom/dad
5	Have a friend over for a play date
6	Choose one toy from toy store
7	Go to miniature golf with family
8	Go to favorite restaurant
10	Go to aquarium with mom/dad

If the Reward Chart and Reward List do not help to motivate your child to read the chapters, you may want to attempt to read your child's book to him. For children with reading disorders or for those who do not like to read, reading to them may be the best option. Give her advance notice that you will help her get started and that the two of you will sit down to read at, for example, 5 p.m. Pick an area of the house that she likes (alternatively, you and your child can go somewhere but most likely it will need to be a place that affords some privacy due to the sensitive topic) and sit down and read to her, suggesting that she help you read some of the chapter, even if it's just a sentence or two. See how it goes; if she quickly becomes open to reading it, you may not need to help her for the remaining chapters; however, if she maintains her disinterest in reading it, I would plan on reading Chapter 2 to her later in the week, then reevaluate.

Occasionally, a child is too young or not at the right point developmentally to be receptive to the program and in this case, waiting for a period of 6 months to a year then trying again may be beneficial. In my clinical practice, I have had several children who were not initially receptive to treatment but when they returned about a year later, they participated very well and successfully overcame their anxiety.

Finally, if the reward system and reading to your child doesn't work and they continue to refuse to read the book, then I would seek additional support, whether it's from your child's pediatrician, the school counselor, or another mental health professional (see References section).

Motivational Strategies for Younger Children Not Willing to Do the Exposures

Many children will have at least some resistance to taking the first step or two on the ladder, so it is best to normalize this for your child. Help her understand that it is normal to feel anxious about taking the first step, yet emphasize that she can handle the feelings of anxiety and now has ways to cope with these feelings and that these feelings generally subside once she is completing her exposures.

If your child maintains that she is unwilling to try the first step, engage in a discussion with her and seek to understand the reasons. Is it possible that the first step on the ladder is actually too hard to be a first step? Is there another step that seems easier or can she think of an easier situation that is not listed on the ladder?

Alternatively, can the first step be broken down into smaller parts to make the tasks more manageable? The key here is to maintain that complete avoidance is no longer an option—she must be willing to try something—and the fact that you are willing to work with her on what that may be shows that you are offering your support and care about her feelings.

Remind your child that he will earn stars on his ladder when he takes a step. (Refer to Chapter 6 for an explanation on how to award stars or stickers). You can emphasize the opportunity to earn rewards and create the Reward List if you haven't already done so.

Motivational Strategies for Early Teens Not Willing to Read the Chapters

Many teens also will respond to a reward program, but may want to document their points earned on a calendar rather than in chart form. Defer to your teen's preferences when it comes to implementing a reward system; your primary role will be approving the appropriateness of their rewards. I find that most teens are very capable of selecting rewards that are appropriate to the points earned, although some have unrealistic expectations and need their parent's assistance in modifying their rewards.

Some young teens will be embarrassed about the program and therefore will reject it. In this case, I recommend that you help reframe the meaning of this program for your teen. Explain that using this program and learning how to overcome his anxiety is a sign of resourcefulness, which is a strong indication of maturity. Highlight the social benefits to overcoming his anxiety, and speak openly that as his parent, you don't want to see him miss out in life because of untreated anxiety. Also, give him permission to keep the fact that he is doing the program private; it is his choice if he wants to share it with others or not.

I caution parents to be careful not to conceptualize seeking professional help as a punishment in any way; seeking professional help is a form of treatment, never a form of punishment. Yet, for teens with anxiety that causes significant impairment in their life, it is only fair that it is calmly explained to them that their anxiety requires treatment, whether it is in the self-help form of this program or with a weekly meeting with mental health professional. Explain that you have selected this program for them as a first step, and while it may be enough for them to overcome their anxiety, additional professional support may be warranted even once they have completed it. Try to explain this in the most loving and supportive way possible.

Motivational Strategies for Early Teens Not Willing to Do the Exposures

As stated above, many children will have at least some hesitation when taking the first step or two on the ladder, so it is best to normalize this for your child. Empathize with your child and explain that it is normal for him to be nervous. The section above, "Motivational Strategies for Younger Children Not Willing to Do the Exposures" applies for teens as well. An additional concern for teens is that they may be more sensitive to the social repercussions of doing exposures. They may be concerned about the fact that they have to do exposures and may feel ashamed about it. In this case, it is helpful to normalize these feelings yet emphasize that the benefits outweigh the costs. You can normalize his feelings by making comments such as, "It makes sense that this is uncomfortable for you—these are things that you have avoided doing for a long time. Taking these steps is supposed to be hard at first," and "The book says that it is normal to feel nervous when facing your fears and the goal is to manage these feelings. You will feel so much better once you get started."

Because one of the primary tasks of adolescence is identity development, it is particularly important to help your early teen develop confidence in himself and his ability to overcome anxiety. One way of promoting this process of confidence development is by not accommodating his anxiety (again this can be accomplished in a gradual manner). Ultimately, this forces your child to deal with the anxiety situation on his own, and this in and of itself will likely serve as a motivator to do the exposures. Once he realizes that you will no longer do the accommodations, he likely will become more motivated to face his fears by doing the exposures. Let me provide a case example:

> Frank was a very bright and very kind 13-year-old boy with OCD. One of his obsessive thoughts involved not killing insects that were in his house; he insisted that they be saved and brought outside of the house. However, he refused to do this himself as he feared coming into contact with the insects. For many years, Frank's family accommodated his anxiety by rescuing various insects (spiders, roaches, moths) from their home, despite their own preference for killing them and flushing them down the toilet. During Frank's treatment with me, we constructed a ladder and included a step on saving bugs on his own. Although he initially protested, he realized that his family would no longer be accommodating him in this way. When it came time to take that step, Frank was able to do it. In fact, he did great! He saved bugs without a problem and even grew comfortable with the idea of killing them from time to time (a rather "normal" event, he learned, as bugs potentially pose a health threat if left to live inside houses). He even reminded his family members that it was up to him to save the bugs. Frank gained confidence in his newfound freedom to take care of the problem on his own, and Frank's family was grateful to no longer have the responsibility of

rescuing bugs found in their house. Frank's identity was now beginning to form out of a sense of confidence and mastery, rather then fear and avoidance.

There are many excellent resources for helping your child be less oppositional and more cooperative, and several of these are listed in the References and Resources sections. If you find that no matter what you try, you still cannot get your child to cooperate, you can offer two choices: that he can complete the program with another (adult) family member or seek professional help. As mentioned in the Introduction, if you do seek professional help, you can request that the therapist use this program with your child (this will be particularly important if the clinician is not very familiar with CBT).

CHAPTER

10
Special Sections

THIS chapter provides additional information and tips on how to help your child depending on which type of anxiety she is experiencing. I recommend reading the section(s) that pertains to your child, as well as the sections at the end on how to handle social situations that are impacted by your child's anxiety (e.g., parties, play dates, explaining the issue to other parents) and how to think about your child's experience with anxiety and the process of overcoming it.

Generalized Anxiety Disorder (GAD)

As mentioned in Chapter 1, children with GAD have excessive worry that is difficult to contain. Their tolerance for stress often is lower than that of other children, and therefore they are more easily overwhelmed. In addition, these children often struggle when it comes to tolerating uncertainty, and this is evidenced by their repetitive questioning of what will happen, what happens if . . . , what the plan will be, how they can be prepared, and so on. Part of

overcoming GAD, then, involves helping them deal with not knowing everything that will or might happen. Dr. Robert Leahy (2006)
wrote a book for adults entitled *The Worry Cure: Seven Steps to Stop
Worry From Stopping You*, which describes a technique called *uncertainty training*. This technique is designed to increase an individual's
tolerance of uncertainty, as well as desensitize the person to his or
her anxiety-provoking thoughts. For example, uncertainty training
involves repeating over and over "It is always possible that . . . "
(e.g., "I might catch a cold," "fail the test," "get in an accident").
With repetition, these anxious thoughts become less alarming and
no longer serve as triggers to experiencing anxiety. Although Dr.
Leahy's book is written for adults, I use uncertainty training with
children and have had a successful outcome. Therefore, in addition
to the strategies that you and your child learned in the previous
chapters, this is another approach that you can teach your child to
use if the other techniques are not enough in helping him control
his worries. By modeling your own tolerance for uncertainty, for
example, with comments like "It is always possible that we will
be late," and "It is always possible that I might get the flu, too,"
you show your child that it is OK not to know everything that
is to come, and that you are happy even without knowing what
might happen in the future. As Dr. Leahy explains, the goal of this
technique is not to neutralize the statement by coming up with a
plan for how you or your child will cope with the uncertain future;
rather, the goal is to become unalarmed by the uncertainty.

Encourage your child to practice uncertainty training and give
her examples on what she can repeat to herself. We do not always
know what will happen in life, and we cannot possibly prepare
ourselves for the future; all we can do is assure ourselves that we
can handle whatever comes our way. It also is a good idea to incorporate exposure to unexpected changes in the schedule into your
child's ladder. For instance, you can recommend including on the
ladder "last minute change in plans," or "mom is late when picking
up the carpool from school" (arrive 10 minutes late, but your child

should not know how late you will be). Alternatively, the step can be "unexpected changes in the plan" and then you can decide last minute to go to a different movie, different restaurant, or have a grandparent drive the carpool for a change. The general idea is for your child to practice things not going exactly as planned, and these opportunities will allow her to realize that unexpected changes are normal. This way, your child will practice stepping outside of his comfort zone.

Because children with GAD usually catastrophize (i.e., expect the worst, visualize disaster) and have excessive worries, it is recommended that you help your child adopt more reality-based thoughts. For example, I worked with an 8-year-old girl who walked by an abandoned gym bag on the sidewalk and worried that "sick germs" could have been in the bag and that when walking by it, she could have caught those germs and gotten sick. I explained to her that bags do not hold sick germs in them and that it is impossible to get sick from walking by a gym bag. This explanation encouraged her to adopt more reality-based patterns of thinking. Children with GAD benefit from being educated about the likelihood of what they worry about actually happening. Sometimes the explanations actually will be reassuring for the child; some reassurance is acceptable in the beginning phases of the program. However, toward later phases, children should be directed to label and replace their thinking errors, such as when they are catastrophizing.

Children with GAD often have symptoms of restlessness, difficulty concentrating, sleep disturbance, and irritability. Children with GAD can seem preoccupied and find it difficult to pay attention; in my experience, some children with GAD have been misdiagnosed with Attention Deficit/Hyperactivity Disorder (ADHD). It is imperative that an ADHD diagnosis is made only after a thorough neuropsychological assessment in which a battery of tests has been administered. In addition, true ADHD doesn't usually improve on its own without medication, whereas GAD may fluctuate in its severity. If your child is anxious and inattentive,

I recommend treating the anxiety first and then reevaluating the inattentiveness. Keep in mind that it is always possible that a child with ADHD also has GAD or has "learning-disorder induced anxiety" (i.e., anxiety from not being able to complete work on time, getting in trouble in school and at home for not paying attention or properly completing tasks).

Finally, children with GAD might require more down time. Overscheduled children with anxiety often can experience relief when their commitments are reduced. I strongly believe that children need at least one day of the weekend when they are not doing any homework and can have time to relax. Recreational time is essential. Similarly, if your child maintains an "I must get all A's" attitude in school, I recommend that "earning a B" on a test or assignment be a step on her ladder. Many children with GAD also are perfectionists and come from high-achievement-oriented families (read the section on perfectionism below). The end goal is to put goals in perspective and ensure that children have time to relax, have downtime, play outside, and opportunities to be creative in a natural, unstructured way. Children benefit from play time and also from having some time to spend alone.

Separation Anxiety Disorder (SAD)

Children with SAD can present parents with quite a challenge, as they often display excessive clinginess or neediness. They often have a limited tolerance for being without a parent and will melt down upon separation. Children with SAD worry about their parent getting hurt or dying. There are varying degrees of this anxiety: Some children constantly seek physical contact with the parent (e.g., a child may hold tightly to his mother's arm) while others may only have difficulty at bedtime and refuse to sleep alone. During the beginning of the treatment process, it is important to reassure your child that by learning how to tolerate being separate, he is not going to be less loved by you, nor will your bond be threatened in any way. In fact, parents may feel less annoyed by their child as he becomes less clingy or learns to sleep alone, and this may allow for more enjoyable time together; however, I would not share this information with your child as it may be hurtful to hear. Comments such as, "I love you all the time, whether I'm with you or not," "It is perfectly safe to sleep alone, and I know you will be OK," and "We are always very close in our hearts, and anytime you want to feel my love for you, just look inside your heart" can be grounding for your child and give him extra support during the ladder practices.

When developing the steps on the ladder, it likely will be necessary to offer smaller steps within each step. For example, let's say that one step is "Mom goes out without you." Your child may need to practice this several times, starting with a 15-minute interval then increasing by 15 minutes until your child can tolerate a 2–3 hour period in which you go out without him. At first, you may make yourself available with a cellular phone, but ultimately your child should be able to do the practice without calling you. It is my assumption that your child is with a trusted adult during these separation practices or is old enough and mature enough to stay at home alone. Your child likely will benefit from the following empathic, supportive statements from you: "I know it feels scary and that you don't like it, but we need to work toward you feeling OK when I go out," "It is important for us to work together to help you feel more comfortable when we're not together," and "I know it might not feel this way now, but you will feel better about yourself once you are able to do this."

Sometimes children develop SAD after they have experienced a trauma, such as a loss of a parent, abuse, or witnessing a violent act. Additionally, some adopted children develop SAD in response to the disruption of, or lack of, a primary caregiver. In these cases, it is important to give the child some time to cope with the trauma or adjust to the new adoptive home, before you begin treating his

SAD. At times, the separation anxiety symptoms are transitory and will resolve on their own as time passes and the child adjusts to the traumatic or stressful situation. However, if symptoms persist after 6–12 months (depending on the event), or if the symptoms worsen in severity, then treatment of the SAD likely is warranted.

Social Phobia (SoP)

Social phobia ranges from mild to severe, and goes beyond discomfort with giving presentations in class, such as oral book reports. Children with social phobia often appear painfully shy and will go to great lengths to avoid social behaviors, such as greeting other children, calling friends, initiating plans, going to parties, and so forth. There are a few thinking errors that are more common to social phobia than the other anxiety disorders, including mind reading and personalization. It will be very helpful for you to point out when your child is making these thinking mistakes. These thinking mistakes can be subtle, such as "I know that my soccer coach doesn't like me," and "My friend cancelled our plans because she is mad at me for not calling her back the other day." It is recommended that you help your child consider other explanations for her coach's or friend's behavior. Additionally, it is important that you do not model being judgmental of others, as the child with social anxiety will use this as evidence that others are judging her as well. For example, commenting that someone on a TV show is "nervous and shaky" gives the cue to your child that others may be making negative judgments about her when she gets up in front of an audience to talk (e.g., book report).

Because social phobia may contribute to a sense of low self-esteem, it is recommended that you challenge your child with questions like, "What would someone who is secure with him- or herself think or do in this situation?" or "How would someone who feels sure about him- or herself handle this?" Challenging thoughts by encouraging your child to consider evidence against her anxious thoughts and predictions is another strategy: "What evidence or proof do you have that this will happen?" Additionally, I recommend that you pay attention to the messages that you give regarding mistakes and failures. It is important to communicate that everyone makes mistakes and that people should be forgiving of themselves when mistakes occur. Similarly, we all do embarrassing things from time to time, and the goal is to foster self-acceptance and forgiveness during these times. Also, children should learn that the cues they give to others regarding their mistakes or embarrassing moments tend to be what others use to know how to respond. For instance, if a child trips and falls in front of others, then gets up and smiles or laughs a bit, others will likely smile or laugh, too.

Several years ago, I was at a wedding and confused a man with the father of the bride; I went on and on complimenting him on the beautiful ceremony, the band, the flowers, how beautiful his daughter looked, and then he corrected me: He wasn't the father of the bride. What an embarrassment! I was so embarrassed and kept playing the scenario over and over in my head, until I finally gave myself a pep-talk and told myself that everyone makes mistakes and this was a nice reminder that I am human and not flawless. I also focused on how well this man handled it: For the rest of the evening, he kept joking with me, calling me "Lonnie, I mean Ronnie," instead of "Bonnie." Should a similarly embarrassing moment occur for you, it offers an opportunity to model how well you handled it: Share the story with your son or daughter and use a sense of humor to show him or her that it's not so bad after all.

An important skill for all children is the skill of assertiveness. Assertiveness, or "sticking up for yourself," differs from aggressiveness as it is respectful of the other person(s) and does not include being physical or forceful. It also differs from being passive (doing nothing) as it is an active behavior. Being assertive is an appropriate, healthy behavior indicative of good self-esteem. When others invade our personal space or discount our personal rights, it is appropriate to respond in an assertive manner. For example, if your child has a friend come over and this friend begins to use her fancy art supplies without asking, it is important that your child be assertive and say, "I'm sorry but you need to ask first before using my paints," or "I am the only one who uses my paints, but I am happy to share my nail polish with you." Although sharing is a positive friendship skill, children also have the right to have their personal space and personal property respected, and it is acceptable to have certain things that are not for sharing.

Because children with social anxiety are oversensitive to being judged negatively by others, they are less likely to be assertive as it incorporates a social behavior that requires confidence and often social risk (e.g., we do not always get the response we'd like). Thus, overcoming social anxiety requires the development of healthy assertive behavior. Parental modeling is an excellent way of showing children how to be assertive. When coaching your child on how to respond in an assertive way, encourage him to maintain good eye contact, stand straight up (no slouching), use a firm, steady voice (not too loud but not soft either), and speak clearly. Nonverbal communication is key; in fact, a classic UCLA study by Albert Mehrabian (Mehrabian & Ferris, 1967) found that 93% of communication is nonverbal (55% through body language and 38% through tone and inflection of voice), so help your child improve his body language, physical presence, and how his voice sounds when being assertive. Initially, you can have discussions with your child *after* the opportunity to be assertive has presented itself and you and your child can discuss how he could have handled the situation in an assertive way. If your child is open to it, you can practice (role-play) the assertive response.

This book does not address in-depth selective mutism, a severe form of Social Phobia characterized by a tendency to refuse to speak with certain people while being completely comfortable speaking fluently with others. The Resources section of this book includes a book on this topic. Finally, it is noted that many children with school refusal/school phobic behavior have an underlying social phobia disorder. Please see the sections below on selective mutism or school refusal if applicable.

Specific Phobia (SP)

Specific phobias can be categorized as "situational type," "animal type," "natural environment type," "blood-injection-injury type," or "other," and again, are differentiated from "fears" as they either involve avoidance of the situations or the situation is tolerated with extreme distress. Situations that often are avoided or intensely feared are flying on planes, going to school (see section below on school refusal), getting sick, and vomiting. Many of the children that I have worked with have the animal type, as they demonstrate an intense fear of dogs, bugs, snakes, spiders, and so forth. The most important advice I give to parents is to show compassion! Having compassion and empathy for your child, even when you don't and can't "get it," is a tremendous gift that you can give. As the nature of a phobia is usually irrational, and the child's reaction to the feared situation is intense and extreme, it is easy for children to feel shamed by their phobia. To prevent this from happening, you can communicate empathy and compassion with comments such as, "I understand how scary this is for you," "I understand how scared you are," and "I know how hard this is for you."

Many parents tell me that they cannot understand why their child cannot just play with a dog, for example. "I don't know what is so bad about a cute harmless dog? Couldn't we just have our daughter play with a dog so she could see that it is OK?" Well-intentioned parents who genuinely want their child to get over the fear make these types of comments. I respond by giving them advice on how to foster and demonstrate empathy. What seems easy to you is excruciatingly painful for them. Although this may be hard to imagine, it may help to consider a time when you felt extremely scared or panicked, for example, if you nearly got in an accident or couldn't find your child in a store, and realize that this is likely your dog-phobic child's experience when he sees a dog.

Depending on the type of phobia your child has, giving him facts or other information about the feared situation can be beneficial. For instance, for children who avoid flying on a plane due to fears of crashing, it would be appropriate to share that, on average, 40,000 people die every year in car accidents whereas only 80 or so die in plane accidents. You do not want to make your child afraid of cars (and typically this will not), but illustrate how we are used to and not afraid of things that are done routinely on a regular, daily basis, such as driving. Also, your child should learn that flying is the safest form of travel and that skilled technicians conduct mechanical tests on each plane before it flies, making it very safe. Turbulence poses no threat to aircraft safety and equates to just a few bumps in the road. A coping plan for flying exposure would include (in addition to relaxation strategies, challenging catastrophic and other thinking errors, and positive self-talk) bringing along a host of distraction activities, such as a book, a deck of cards, a music player, a stuffed animal, and puzzles. Self-talk for flying examples include: "Flying is the safest form of travel and I will be fine," "Turbulence is normal and safe," "Once we have taken off, I will get used to flying and feel comfortable," and "I have a lot of things that I will do to distract myself. I always feel better when I listen to music." Similarly, children who are afraid of dogs should learn that most dogs are harmless and won't bite, although there are certain techniques to use when approaching a dog, such as asking the owner if the dog is safe to touch, approaching the dog slowly but confidently, cupping your hand in front of and below the dog's mouth/nose, and letting the dog sniff you first. Providing this step-by-step structure often is grounding for the child with phobias and offers her a planned out approach to working through the situation.

Obsessive-Compulsive Disorder (OCD)

Obsessive-compulsive disorder is a little different from the other anxiety disorders in childhood. First of all, it can be very subtle. I am always amazed at how hidden the symptoms can be, and many parents share my amazement. For example, children may walk in a certain way, so as to avoid cracks on the sidewalk or walk in a symmetrical fashion (e.g., left foot first in the first square on the block, then right foot first in the second square; or, left side of foot touches rim of square on the sidewalk then right side of foot touches the opposite rim), or do a variety of subtle behaviors that often are missed by others around them. For these reasons, giving your child permission to discuss the rituals and creating an open environment to do so is crucial. I find that children respond when I am confident during the inquiry process, "So, I know bathrooms are hard for you—do you avoid touching the flusher, toilet seat, stall lock, faucet, and bathroom door handle?" I make it known that it is usually pervasive (covers a lot of behaviors in the anxiety situation) and that many rituals are involved in OCD. Most parents can identify many of the rituals that their child performs and this is a great start, but 9 times out of 10, there are many, many more rituals that go unnoticed by parents.

Sometimes children can have a form of OCD in which there are no explicit or observable behaviors but just a mental experience, referred to as *Pure-O*. It used to be thought that individuals with Pure-O only had obsessive thoughts; however, it is now understood that there often are mental acts or mental compulsions that children do in response to the obsessive thoughts. For example, a client of mine with Pure-O would get mentally stuck on a very specific and irrelevant component of a math equation and in response to the obsessive thoughts about it, she would run through the equation over and over for hours until it "felt right." This goes beyond simply obsessive thinking, is incredibly time-consuming, and results in an impairment of some kind such as difficulty focusing in class or when conversing with others.

Children with OCD often are perfectionistic as well as obsessive-compulsive and this perfectionism may or may not be part of the OCD. See the section on perfectionism below for more information. All-or-nothing thinking and catastrophizing also are commonly seen in children with OCD.

There are a few additional thinking errors specific to OCD (all explained in the book by Hyman described below), including "thought-action fusion," "superstitious thinking," and "overimportance of thoughts." Depending on your child's age, you may or may not choose to discuss these with him. Listed below are definitions and examples of each:

- ► **Thought-Action Fusion:** If I think something, then it will happen or may have happened. When thinking this way, there is no difference between thinking you did something and believing you actually did it.
  Example: "If I think about lighting the candle, then I better check to make sure it has not been lit or to blow it out."
  Example: "If I think about hurting my brother then I better check that he is OK and unharmed."
- ► **Superstitious Thinking:** By thinking or doing something, I will cause or prevent something else from happening.
  Example: "If I wash my hands 33 times a day, then my parents will be safe."
  Example: "If I knock twice with my left hand and twice with my right hand and say a prayer, nothing bad with happen to me."
- ► **Overimportance of Thoughts:** My thoughts describe my true feelings. Thinking certain thoughts says something bad about me. Thoughts have a lot of meaning associated with them.

Example: "If I have the intrusive thought that we will drive off the bridge, then it means that I want us all to die."
Example: "If I have a sexual thought about my friend, then I am a pervert."

Bruce Hyman, Ph.D., author of *The OCD Workbook: Your Guide to Breaking Free From Obsessive-Compulsive Disorder* (Hyman & Pedrick, 2005), written for adults, summarizes the OCD cycle. The four parts of the cycle (in order) are: "(1) activating event, (2) unrealistic appraisal of the event, (3) excessive anxiety, and (4) neutralizing ritual" (Hyman & Pedrick, 2005, p. 100). Let me go through a few examples, using the numbers to identify the steps:

▶ (1) use a public restroom, (2) obsessive thought that restrooms have many bad germs and that these bad germs will get on me and I will get sick or will get cancer, (3) very anxious, and (4) wash hands thoroughly with lots of soap;

▶ (1) walk by an abandoned bag on the street, (2) irrational thought that the bag has toxic airborne substance in it, (3) very anxious, and (4) ask mom over and over for reassurance that I did not get sick from passing bag on street.

▶ (1) walking on sidewalk, (2) obsessive thought that if I step with my left foot in the square then I need step with my right foot in the same square, (3) very anxious, and (4) must step with both left foot and right foot in each square.

Understanding the OCD cycle helps your child externalize the OCD and can give him greater awareness of his experience with OCD. I recommend teaching your child about the cycle and going through a few examples with him.

Children do not need to recognize the irrationality of their obsessive thoughts in order to be diagnosed with OCD (whereas adults do need to recognize it). It often is the case where a child lacks insight into his or her OCD and does not question the meaning or relevance of it. OCD also can appear as very odd behavior, such as hoarding trash or food under one's bed, touching one's ear in a repetitive way, or walking in and out of a room over and over. Most parents have a difficult time truly "getting" the severity of the urge or pull that a compulsion causes. I recommend that, as much as possible, you should show compassion for your child and try to manage the normal frustrations that come from witnessing your child's odd and pointless behavior.

Compared to the other anxiety disorders, there seems to be more of a genetic component with OCD. For this reason, I often will recommend that the child be evaluated for medication (typically an SSRI) if the OCD thoughts continue to persist after 3 months (or 12–14 sessions) of CBT. However, it is important to keep in mind that research shows that children and adults with OCD who are treated only with medication and not CBT or other therapy do not do nearly as well as those who have CBT treatment, whether that treatment occurs alone without medication or in addition to medication.

Panic Disorder (PD)

The most important first step in helping a child who suffers from panic attacks is teaching her to label the panic attack itself. Labeling it and teaching your child the symptoms of panic is incredibly beneficial, as it helps normalize what is happening and this will allow your child to relax and learn not to have a secondary panic attack about the fact that she is panicking. Initially, you will label the panic attack for her and then reassure your child that she can handle it and that the panic attack will pass (no one in the history of the world has ever stayed stuck in a panic attack!). In fact, accepting it typically will cause it to pass in a shorter time. However, once your child has completed the program, you simply will help her label the panic attack and encourage her to reassure herself (e.g., asking "What do you think is going on for you right now?" cues her that it is panic). It is noteworthy that many children with panic attacks are sensitive to minor changes in their bodies, such as shortness of breath, thus it will be helpful for you to explain that there are normal fluctuations in the body and that these changes are not of concern.

Ultimately, your child needs to be encouraged to "ride the wave" of panic. This in and of itself actually will lessen the severity of the panic. He or she needs to learn to be able to tolerate and not fear the symptoms. Panic is a frightening experience and it becomes worsened by the worry that one is panicking: The child with panic is most anxious about the fact that he is panicking—it truly is a "fear of fear." The panic attack itself is not threatening or damaging, but simply very, very uncomfortable and unpleasant. By knowing what is happening and knowing that one can handle it and that it will pass, the panic can become less severe.

One way in which I work with children on the goal of not being afraid of the symptoms of panic attacks is actually to practice the symptoms with them. Although most of the research on this strategy has been conducted with adults, I have found this method to work with most school-age children. Even if they don't get very anxious when practicing the symptoms, it is effective because they get the message: I don't have to be afraid of panic. To practice the symptoms, I have children deliberately "hyperventilate" (breathe in and out rapidly and loudly) and allow them to tolerate the discomfort (once we complete this exercise and they have been able to handle the uncomfortable feelings, then I will do calm breathing to get them back to a normal baseline). Other ways of inducing symptoms include running and up and down the stairs (rapid heartbeat) and then turning around in circles (dizziness), or breathing in and out through a very small straw (difficulty breathing). Practicing the symptoms can be included on their ladder, as this is how they are facing their fears: "Practice anxious breathing," "Practice feeling dizzy," "Practice having a fast heartbeat." A great reference on this approach is *Facing Panic* by R. Reid Wilson

(2003; available at http://www.adaa.org). Originally written for adults, I successfully apply the concepts of this book to my work with children.

Like OCD, panic attacks occur in a cycle. R. Reid Wilson (2003) does a fantastic job of explaining the cycle, which has four parts: "(1) anticipatory anxiety, (2) panic attack, (3) escape and relief, and (4) self-doubt and self-criticism" (p. 6). Not all children with panic necessarily go though these four stages, but the cycle describes what many experience. The anticipatory anxiety (e.g., "Oh, no! What if I panic?") increases a child's anxiety level and he worries about an impending panic attack, which increases the likelihood of a panic attack. Once the panic attack occurs, the idea of leaving the situation is linked with feeling a strong sense of relief. Following this escape/relief, an experience of self-doubt and feeling badly about oneself comes up. For example, I worked with a child who would get anxious about going to school. He would work himself up into a panic attack (it always started with anticipatory anxiety the night before a school day, but was particularly worse in the morning and once he arrived at school). By first period, he would be in a full-blown panic attack and would go to the school nurse who promptly called his mother (at his request) to pick him up. His mother, a warm and loving woman who had genuine concern for her child's health, quickly came to school and inadvertently reinforced (and worsened) his anxiety. Once he was home, he would feel embarrassed and "like a failure" because he couldn't stay in school. During his treatment with me, he learned that he needed to stay in school no matter what—even if he needed to take a break from classes to go to the nurse's office—he needed to return to class once he felt a bit calmer. The most important goals are (1) not panicking about panicking, and (2) not avoiding activities or situations because of a fear of panic or a panic attack itself.

Tips on Other Anxiety-Driven Behaviors or Problems

Perfectionism

Perfectionism often is a developmentally appropriate characteristic in childhood: Children are socialized to understand that there is a right way and a wrong way to do things, that things should be done in a certain order, that they should clean up after themselves, and so on. This type of learning is appropriate and necessary. Therefore, children can show perfectionistic traits when attempting to "follow the rules." However, there comes a time when flexibility and the ability to consider alternatives to the usual way of doing things becomes important, and essential. If a child does not grow and evolve in this way, she may get "stuck in" a state of perfectionism. When this happens, children display rigidity and inflexibility, resulting in frustration and unhappiness.

Perfectionistic children often have to have things a certain way in order to feel OK, and typically have a hard time accepting that there is more than one way to do something. For example, they tend to be overly concerned with the right and wrong and insist that things be done in the "right" way. A child who spends 3 hours on a math assignment that should take no more than 45 minutes because he needs to check and recheck his work is demonstrating extreme perfectionism. Another, less extreme example is the child who exhibits significant distress over earning a B on a quiz in a class where she has mostly A's on her work, and may cry or throw a tantrum as a result. These rigid and inflexible approaches to dealing with life events should be challenged in the same spirit as the other anxiety behaviors are challenged. Thus, they should be integrated into the child's ladder and practiced in the same way. For instance, a step on the ladder could be "get a B on a quiz on purpose," "miss the bus one day," or "check over your work only once and stop working after 1 hour." These examples give perfectionistic children the experience of learning that things will work out for them, even if they are not done in the "right" or "best" or "usual" way. The practices also help to, as my good colleague Dr. Charlie Manseuto says, "Welcome the child to the world of the 'good enough.'" For example, children who must have everything excessively organized in their room at all times at the expense of having play time learn that they could skip putting every single thing away in its place and leave a part of the room temporarily cluttered and play with their neighbor instead of cleaning. When it comes to keeping their room a certain way, they learn that they can be "good enough" about it with no repercussions.

Challenging the child's perfectionistic thoughts also is important. All-or-nothing thinking and "shoulds" tend to organize the child's cognitive life in addition to how he behaves. Helping children learn to replace these thoughts with healthier, more balanced thoughts is part of the process of change. In the Resources section, I have included a book called *When Perfect Isn't Good Enough* by Martin Antony and Richard Swinson. This book provides excellent descriptions of the common perfectionistic thoughts and behaviors and although it is written for adults (and older teens), it certainly applies to the understanding of perfectionism in children, and parents will benefit from reviewing it (although it would need to be verbally adapted for children to understand). As stated above, perfectionism sometimes can be a symptom of OCD, and the book's authors include a chapter on this link.

Being Easily Overwhelmed

Many anxious children get overwhelmed easily, and this tendency to be overwhelmed often centers on school—schoolwork, homework, and tests. If your child experiences this, try helping her develop the daily behavior of creating "To do" checklists, in which she lists out the subjects and the homework in each. Help her to be "in the moment," and only focus on the task at hand. For example you can make her a self-talk note card that reads: "I need to be in the present moment and only focus on one thing at a time," or "When I only focus on the assignment I am working on, I am OK." Uncertainty training (described above under the GAD section) also can be used for this issue; for example, your child can practice repeating: "It is always possible that I won't finish all of my work." With repetition, scary thoughts will be neutralized and will no longer create a feeling of anxiety.

You might need to monitor her approach to doing her homework and help her organize the assignments, perhaps breaking down assignments into smaller steps so they seem more manageable. When you see your child becoming overwhelmed, encourage her to take a 10-minute break to calm down and then return to doing her work with a more relaxed attitude. If this can be done repetitively, your child will soon begin to associate doing homework with being calm. Otherwise, if your child continues to focus on her work while her heart is beating and she is rushing and nervous, she will associate homework with being anxious.

Many children experience test anxiety. This can cause a huge interference for your child, and may even cause your child to blank out and not score as well on exams. Relaxation techniques, uncertainty training, challenging catastrophic thinking, and creating steps on the ladder to expose your child to test situations will help your child overcome his test anxiety. The ladder exposures can include: practice tests at home, practice timed tests at home, working collaboratively with teachers to let your child take a pretest (a test before the real test on similar content area), and deliberately getting a few items on a test wrong (use for extremely perfectionistic children who expect to get every item correct and all A's on every test and have test anxiety as a result).

Finally, it can be helpful to use a calendar and stickers to note each day that your child approaches his homework in a calm and collected way. This provides a way to track his progress and also redefines success as being calm and relaxed and puts the focus on the approach taken toward doing homework, rather than the focus on finishing all of the work perfectly.

Excessive Guilt

Some children, most of whom have generalized anxiety and many of whom are perfectionistic, exhibit the symptom of excessive guilt. Although the emotion of guilt can be useful in that it represents one's conscience and keeps the person "in check" with his or her values, *excessive* guilt serves no purpose, other than to make the person feel miserable. Children who have excessive guilt may repeatedly say, "I feel bad," and get triggered into feeling guilty (and often anxious) from meaningless events. For example, Melissa, a bright and very kind 13-year-old, felt bad every time her parents bought her something. She needed new cleats for soccer and when simply reminding her mother that she needed them, she was triggered into hours-long feelings of guilt. Sometimes she would feel so bad that she would cry. As a typical teenager, Melissa enjoyed getting new things and appreciated dressing nicely; however, this enjoyment was compromised by her contrasting feelings of excessive guilt. What should have been a pleasurable experience became a source of much distress and unhappiness. In this way, Melissa's guilt caused an interference in her life. In the course of her treatment with me, Melissa shared tons of things that made her feel guilty, such as forgetting to say goodnight to her babysitter, being annoyed with one of her classmates (a common experience for everyone), going shopping with her parents, and getting a reward from her mother for reading a book.

Melissa and I identified her thinking errors, which included "shoulds" ("I should never forget to say goodnight to the babysitter," "I should not have nice things when there are all these poor people in the world"), and then made a cassette tape recording (over two sessions—doing it on 2 different days was very helpful) of *everything* she felt guilty or bad about. I instructed her to listen to the tape over and over for at least 15 minutes each day. Within a month of doing this, Melissa's guilty thoughts went away, and they stayed away! Several months later, she even commented with both surprise and excitement, "I don't feel bad anymore!" The excitement in her voice reflected her newfound freedom. When children feel bad and anxious, they are robbed of the freedom to simply enjoy life. Gaining freedom from this, and a stronger sense of confidence about herself and her feelings, was liberating for Melissa.

If your child experiences excessive guilt, you also can make a tape with him of all of the things that he feels guilty about and then play the tape repeatedly like Melissa did. The main goal of the tape is twofold: (1) to help your child externalize his emotions, taking the emotion from inside his mind to outside of himself and (2) to help him *habituate*, or become used to his guilt-provoking or distressing thoughts. Finally, it is beneficial to make your child some self-talk note cards on this subject. Some examples include: "Feelings are not right or wrong or good or bad. I will not feel bad about my feelings," "Feeling guilty when I did not do anything wrong is useless," and "Everyone makes mistakes. No one is perfect, including me."

Health Anxiety

Children with health anxiety include those who are hyper-focused on physical symptoms, preoccupied with a health issue, complain of something wrong with their health, and those who often want medical help or treatment. Although health anxiety most often is a part of either GAD or OCD, it can be a problem in and of itself. Initially, I refer these children for a comprehensive physical exam to rule out true medical problems. I recommend the medical exam for two reasons: (1) children with health anxiety get sick and have medical problems just as children without health anxiety do, and (2) this allows me to refer to fact-based evidence that they are healthy and this is really only anxiety, so that I can treat the "symptoms" as anxiety symptoms.

The best recommendation I can make to parents is to offer as much compassion as possible without enabling the child (e.g., allowing the child to miss school or other obligations) and accommodating the fears or reinforcing the health anxiety (e.g., repeatedly bringing him to different doctors, giving him reassurance, letting him sleep in your bed when he is complaining of not feeling well). Whether or not there is a real problem and whether or not your child consciously is using physical complaints in a manipulative way, your child is struggling with feeling OK. The balance is responding to this struggle and her worries in a caring and loving way without reinforcing her beliefs and behaviors. Working with her to identify if there is something stressful that is upsetting her and promoting a proactive (versus reactive) response can be a good start. Proactive means taking an active approach that is problem solving and rational, not emotion-driven. For example, coaching your child to find activities that are distracting or enjoyable to cope with feeling ill or worrying about symptoms teaches her to be proactive, whereas the reactive response includes crying, complaining, and checking for symptoms.

Hair Pulling

Hair pulling, called *trichotillomania* or trich for short, is a repetitive behavior disorder in which the individual pulls hair from her head or scalp, eyebrows, eyelashes, or other parts of her body. This is distinguished from other "picking" habits such as nail biting or picking skin, as it is exclusive to hair and also more complex. The hair pulling behavior can feel like an addiction and there is a tactile (touch) sensation to the pulling of the hair that is strongly reinforced each time the child pulls. Bald spots or missing eyebrows or lashes are common and this can cause the person to feel socially embarrassed. Hair pulling is best treated with professional help. As it is beyond the scope of this book, I have provided resources in the Resources section for this topic.

School Refusal Behavior

School refusal behavior can be a symptom of severe social phobia and tends to cause a significant interference that can go on for years and cause tremendous distress for the child and the whole family. Alternatively, school refusal can be a form of oppositional defiant disorder (ODD; see the Resources section for books on defiant or explosive children). Although this topic is not a focal point of the book, I will make a few suggestions based on my work with this population of children. Frankly, this is one of the most challenging problems to address but I have worked with many successful cases so I encourage you to stay hopeful about a solution to this problem.

First and foremost, the child's school and parents need to be involved in addressing this problem. There needs to be a contact person at the child's school who is willing to check in daily with the parents and whom the child will report to when she attends school or when she does not (e.g., call from home). When there is a therapist involved in the treatment process, that therapist should work closely with the school as well. If possible, a multidisciplinary team meeting with the parents, therapist, school counselor/teachers/principal, and possibly the child (depending on the age—children 10 and above should attend and younger children can, as well, although there should be some discussion about it), should be arranged at the school.

Second, parents will need to alter their parenting approach around the subject of school attendance and discipline. School refusal behavior typically includes an oppositional component and many children with this issue also meet the criteria for an oppositional defiant disorder. Researchers have identified four types of parenting styles, all described by the amount of warmth and the amount of demand/expectations that parents place upon their children (Baumrind, 1991; Maccoby & Martin, 1983). The four types and descriptions are as follows, going from most demand placed on the child to least demand placed on the child but not in order of rank: authoritarian (high demand, low warmth), authoritative (high demand, high warmth), permissive (low demand, high warmth), and uninvolved (low demand, low warmth). The type that has been found to be the best is the authoritative type (high demand, high warmth); these are parents who are empathic and sensitive to their child's emotions and offer warmth and concern, yet they have expectations for their child and will provide appropriate and reasonable discipline and consequences when these expectations are not met. The type that I find occurs most often in families with children who refuse to attend school is the permissive type. When working with these families, I typically do separate sessions with the parent(s) and help them develop an attitude of expectations and authority while maintaining empathy and warmth. Too many children in these families believe that it is their *choice* to attend or not to attend school. Scott Sells, author of *Parenting Your Out-of-Control Teenager: 7 Steps to Reestablish Authority and Reclaim Love* (2002), identifies that one of the biggest problems is unclear rules. Many families with school refusal children do not communicate the rule that children must attend school, and that attending school is nonnegotiable. The message parents need to give is that attending school is not an option—it is a rule! Just as adults have to go to work, children need to go to school—it is their job. And, just as adults who choose not to go to work suffer the consequences (e.g., no money, no new clothes, no entertainment), children who choose not to go to school also should have these consequences (of course, removal of food and/or shelter should never be included in these consequences).

Third, learning disabilities (LD) or learning differences need to be considered as contributing factors in a child's refusal to go to school. Some children with school refusal have underlying dyslexia or auditory processing problems that make it hard for them to understand what they are learning and do the work in the time allotted. It might be necessary to have your child tested for learning differences. If he has an LD, the school is required to create an IEP (Individualized Education Program) for your child, giving him the accommodations he needs to attain academic success.

Fourth, what initially caused the school refusal behavior and what maintains it may not be the same. Once a significant amount of school has been missed, the child loses his sense of belonging in the school and typically feels lost in the classroom and isolated socially. I recommend that you give your child assurance that once he returns to school on a daily (thus, consistent) basis, these issues will dissolve. He will catch up academically (ideally, the school will make some accommodations and reduce the amount of make-up work) and he will improve socially. The most important idea for your child to grasp is that there is only one solution: to go to school! This problem will not be resolved and will not go away until he goes to school on time every day.

Finally, there are two different theories that apply to school refusal. The first is choice theory created by William Glasser (1998), which explains that we are responsible for the actions we take, and we are responsible for solving our problems. Choice theory also explains that we choose our thoughts, and this is consistent with CBT. Glasser explains that there are four basic psychological needs: "love and belonging, power, freedom, and fun" (p. 28). Your child will have an incredibly challenging time getting these needs met if she is not doing her job of attending school. By not attending school, she loses the need of belonging and love by friends and teachers. She becomes disempowered by not being able to overcome her anxiety about attending. By losing privileges for not going to school (which should be happening), she loses her sense of freedom and cannot have fun.

The second theory is about motivation and success. *Mindset: The New Psychology of Success* by Carol Dweck (2006) explains that there are two types of mindsets: the fixed and the growth. Most people have a combination of both in general, but usually lean closer to one when approaching challenging tasks. In the fixed mindset, people believe that they are born with a certain amount of intelligence, talent, and ability. This is fixed and therefore, cannot be changed. Thus, these individuals spend their lives proving their intelligence, talent, and ability, and if they do not "get" something immediately, they assume it's outside of their range of ability and do not try to learn it. They believe that effort is a sign of failure because if you have to try at it, you are not good at it. In the growth mindset, on the other hand, people believe that while they are born with a certain amount of intelligence, talent, and ability, at any time they can become more intelligent and develop talents and new abilities by putting forth effort and persisting at learning. These individuals approach challenges with perseverance, and believe that effort will equal success. Clearly, the growth mindset is the one to encourage, and Dweck's book includes a section for parents on how to instill the growth mindset in children. Much of her research is done on fifth graders, and there is a good argument to make about developing the growth mindset in childhood for a more successful experience in adulthood. It may be possible that your child has a learning issue or doesn't feel capable of succeeding in school, and that a fixed mindset is interfering with his ability to cope with and overcome these problems or fears.

Selective Mutism

As stated above, selective mutism is not addressed in-depth in this book (see the Resources section for recommended books on this topic). Selective mutism is a less common form of Social Phobia in which the child refuses to speak in certain circumstances (e.g., in particular situations or when around specific people) but speaks freely and openly, often in an extroverted way, in other circumstances. For example, a child with selective mutism may remain completely silent at school and avoid all eye contact but once at home, she will brighten up and speak freely in a loud voice, often openly stating opinions and preferences. One misconception about children with selective mutism is that, because they are not talking, they are not communicating. On the contrary, these children communicate quite a bit nonverbally. One child I worked with who had selective mutism did not speak to me at all for eight sessions, yet, starting at the fourth meeting, she brought in artwork and dolls to show me and her eye contact gradually increased. Although these children can be painfully slow to warm up to new people and become comfortable in new situations, research supports a CBT approach with systematic desensitization (using the step-by-step ladder exposures as a guide).

PTSD

Post-Traumatic Stress Disorder (PTSD) is classified as an anxiety disorder, although it typically involves a trauma or loss that requires specialized treatment (e.g., therapy for sexual or physical abuse, grief therapy). For this reason, and because it most likely requires professional intervention, it is not included in the scope of this book.

Bedwetting

Bedwetting sometimes can be a manifestation of anxiety, although it often is not caused by anxiety. If your child is wetting, it is important to consult with your pediatrician and rule out any physical problems before psychological causes are considered. Regardless of the causes, under no circumstances should children be shamed or criticized for wetting the bed. However, children can be involved in either cleaning up after the wetting or assisting in the clean-up, as this can (but does not always) reduce his embarrassment because he took part in remedying the situation. Please refer to a book on this subject listed in the Resources section for more information.

Tips on Handling Your Child's Anxiety With Others

Another issue that comes up for parents of children with anxiety is how to handle informing others of the anxiety problem. This includes what to say to other parents and children; managing play dates, parties, and sleepovers; and working with other parents when their own child becomes part of the exposure practice (e.g., if one of your child's steps on the ladder is to have a sleepover).

Other parents generally will be understanding when you explain that your child has an anxiety problem; remember that all children experience anxiety at some point in their lives. The more factual you are, the better. Explain that your child has anxiety about _____ (separation, social events, sleepovers, dogs), and that you and your child are working on this problem. Explain that you are arranging "practices" for him to learn how to face his fears, and that you would really appreciate their support.

For example, let's say that your child has either separation anxiety or social anxiety and is invited to a sleepover party. Talking with the parent who is throwing the party is necessary. Once you explain about the anxiety, tell the other parent that your child has strategies that he can use, such as calm breathing and positive self-talk, and that while he may be anxious at first, he will become comfortable soon. If the other parent is comfortable (and you trust that he or she can handle it), he or she can tell your child, "I spoke with your mom (or dad) and I know that you are working on feeling better about sleepovers. If you are having a hard time, please let me know." This gives your child the sense that there is someone else who is temporarily on her team and who can offer support if needed. The other parent should know that if your child does approach him or her, any discussion of your child's anxiety should occur in private. You can make a plan with your child and the other parent that if it becomes too hard for your child, he can give a cue to the other parent and together they can call you for additional support. Your child should know that while he is strongly discouraged from leaving the sleepover (as this can strengthen the avoidance behavior), in a worst-case scenario, you will come and pick him up. The reason for this is that no child should be *forced* to do any of the exposures, as this can make her even more anxious to face her fears and reinforce a sense of disempowerment or helplessness. During the exposure practice, she needs to know that she has a way out of a scary situation if it becomes too much for her to handle. Usually, most ladders should include several gradual steps for sleepovers, such as going to the party but leaving just before bedtime. Again, while I do not condone fibbing or lying, I think it is perfectly reasonable that your child have the option of keeping the fact that he is facing his fears a private matter. Thus, making up excuses while doing the ladder should be an option. For instance, in the case where your child leaves before bedtime, he can tell the other children that he has a family event the next day that requires him to get up really early to attend, and so he needs to sleep at home. Also, if he needs to leave early, he can make the excuse that he is not feeling well. This helps to prevent feeling further isolated from peers and additionally stressed about what to say. As a general rule, the more you plan out the exposure, including preparing your child for what he could say in a variety of different scenarios, the better off you (and he!) will be.

Sometimes your child will show signs of anxiety while in the presence of other children, for example, when on a play date. The same recommendation to be factual applies and you can say, "Sally has a phobia of dogs, which means she is afraid of them, but she is working to get rid of it. I know it might be hard to understand since you love dogs, but some kids are very afraid of them." With anxiety disorders other than phobias, it is best to *describe* the symptom rather than using the terms "obsessive-compulsive disorder" or "separation anxiety disorder." For instance, you can say, "Sometimes Ruth gets nervous about sharing food with other people, but she is working on it," or "Sometimes Thelma has a hard time doing things alone, but she is working on it." This helps to describe the behavior and identify it as a problem that is being addressed. I recommend that this approach be used with friends of your child and not simply acquaintances or children that may tease others. Most children will appreciate the clarification and not question it.

One Last Thought for Parents

First, I want to congratulate you again for taking this important and proactive step of helping your child with his anxiety. As a parent, it is extremely painful to watch your child experience hurt and discomfort, which is generally part of the picture with an anxious child. Many parents worry about being responsible for their child's anxiety disorder, and feel conflicted about how to handle it—swaying between an instinct to comfort and soothe their child and a desire to challenge him and make him stronger. The purpose of this book has been to give you guidance on how to best manage this fine line and how to help your child overcome his fears. Even if you end up needing professional support to treat your child's anxiety, starting with this book is something to be proud of. I also want to reassure you that, while anxiety can have genetic influences, the majority of parents have not caused their child to be anxious. Although modeling anxious responses has been found to be a possible contributor to the development of anxiety, most of the time it simply "just shows up" as a problem.

Overcoming anxiety, as delineated in this program, can foster resilience in children, as they learn how to problem solve, face difficult situations, and take a proactive approach. On a personal note, dealing with and working through my own childhood experience of loss and the resulting separation anxiety helped prepare me for the future and made me stronger and more resilient. Obviously, it also made me a believer in therapy and self-help! Not only do children benefit from overcoming their fears, but they often are more therapy-friendly as they have either completed this program as a "self-help" approach led by me, a psychologist, or in the context of a therapeutic relationship with a mental health professional. Being familiar with therapy in childhood can make it easier to use it as a resource or reference in adulthood.

References

Barlow, D. (2004). Psychological treatments. *American Psychologist, 59,* 869–878.

Baumrind, D. (1991). The influence of parenting style on adolescent competence and substance use. *Journal of Early Adolescence, 11,* 56–95.

Christophersen, E. R., & Mortweet, S. L. (2001). *Treatments that work with children: Empirically supported strategies for managing childhood problems.* Washington, DC: American Psychological Association.

Costello, E. J., & Angold, A. (1995). Epidemiology. In J. March (Ed.), *Anxiety disorders in children and adolescents* (pp. 109–124). New York: Guilford Press.

Curry, J. F., March, J. S., & Hervey, A. S. (2004). Comorbidity of childhood and adolescent anxiety disorders. In T. H. Ollendick & J. S. March (Eds.), *Phobic and anxiety disorders in children and adolescents: A clinician's guide to effective psychosocial and pharmacological interventions* (pp. 116–140). New York: Oxford University Press.

Dweck, C. (2006). *Mindset: The new psychology of success.* New York: Random House.

Glasser, W. (1998). *Choice theory: A new psychology of personal freedom.* New York: HarperPerennial.

Hollon, S. D., Stewart, M. O., & Strunk, D. (2006). Enduring effects for cognitive behavior therapy in the treatment of depression and anxiety. *Annual Review of Psychology, 57,* 285–315.

Hyman, B. M., & Pedrick, C. (2005). *The OCD workbook: Your guide to breaking free from obsessive-compulsive disorder* (2nd ed.). Oakland, CA: New Harbinger.

Jensen, P. S., Hinshaw, S. P., Kraemer, H. C., Lenora, N., Newcorn, J. H., Abikoff, H. B., et al. (2001). ADHD comorbidity findings from the MTA study: Comparing comorbid subgroups. *Journal of the American Academy of Child & Adolescent Psychiatry, 40,* 147–158.

Leahy, R. L. (2006). *The worry cure: Seven steps to stop worry from stopping you.* New York: Harmony Books.

Maccoby, E. E., & Martin, J. A. (1983). Socialization in the context of the family: Parent-child interaction. In P. H. Mussen (Ed.) & E. M. Hetherington (Vol. Ed.), *Handbook of child psychology: Vol. 4: Socialization, personality, and social development* (4th ed., pp. 1–101). New York: Wiley.

Mehrabian, A., & Ferris, S. R. (1967). Inference of attitudes from nonverbal communication in two channels. *Journal of Consulting Psychology, 31,* 248–252.

Sells, S. P. (2002). *Parenting your out-of-control teenager: 7 steps to reestablish authority and reclaim love.* New York: St. Martin's Griffin.

Shaffer, D., Fisher, P., Dulcan, M. K., Davies, M., Piacentini, J., Schwab-Stone, M. E., et al. (1996). The NIMH Diagnostic Interview Schedule for Children Version 2.3 (DISC-2.3): Description, acceptability, prevalence rates, and performance in the MECA study. *Journal of the American Academy of Child & Adolescent Psychiatry, 35,* 865–877.

Vanzant, I. (1998). *One day my soul just opened up.* New York: Fireside.

Wilson, R. R. (2003). *Facing panic: Self-help for people with panic attacks.* Silver Spring, MD: Anxiety Disorders Association of America.

Resources for Parents

Recommended Books and Articles for Parents and Professionals

General Anxiety

Bourne, E. J. (2005). *The anxiety & phobia workbook* (4th ed.). Oakland, CA: New Harbinger.

Chansky, T. (2004). *Freeing your child from anxiety: Powerful, practical solutions to overcome your child's fears, worries, and phobias.* New York: Broadway Books.

Dacey, J. S., & Fiore, L. B. (2000). *Your anxious child: How parents and teachers can relieve anxiety in children.* San Francisco: Jossey-Bass.

Davis, M., Eshelman, E. R., & McKay, M. (2000). *The relaxation & stress reduction workbook* (5th ed.). Oakland, CA: New Harbinger.

Last, C. G. (2006). *Help for worried kids: How your child can conquer anxiety & fear.* New York: Guilford Press.

Leahy, R. L. (2006). *The worry cure: Seven steps to stop worry from stopping you.* New York: Harmony Books.

Rapee, R. M., Spence, S. H., Cobham, V., & Wignall, A. (2000). *Helping your anxious child: A step-by-step guide for parents.* Oakland, CA: New Harbinger.

Separation Anxiety

Eisen, A. R., & Engler, L. B. (2006). *Helping your child overcome separation anxiety or school refusal: A step-by-step guide for parents.* Oakland, CA: New Harbinger.

Eisen, A. R., & Schaefer, C. E. (2005). *Separation anxiety in children and adolescents: An individualized approach to assessment and treatment.* New York: Guilford Press.

Social Anxiety

Antony, M. M., & Swinson, R. P. (2008). *The shyness and social anxiety workbook: Proven step-by-step techniques for overcoming your fears* (2nd ed.). Oakland, CA: New Harbinger.

Carducci, B. J. (2000). *Shyness: A bold new approach*. New York: Harper.

Specific Phobias

Antony, M. M., & McCabe, R. E. (2005). *Overcoming animal & insect phobias: How to conquer fear of dogs, snakes, rodents, bees, spiders, & more*. Oakland, CA: New Harbinger.

Antony, M. M., & Rowa, K. (2007). *Overcoming fear of heights: How to conquer acrophobia & live a life without limits*. Oakland, CA: New Harbinger.

Antony, M. M., & Watling, M. A. (2006). *Overcoming medical phobias: How to conquer fear of blood, needles, doctors, and dentists*. Oakland, CA: New Harbinger.

OCD

Hyman, B. M., & Pedrick, C. (2005). *The OCD workbook: Your guide to breaking free from obsessive-compulsive disorder* (2nd ed.). Oakland, CA: New Harbinger.

Wagner, A. P. (2002). *What to do when your child has obsessive-compulsive disorder: Strategies and solutions*. Rochester, NY: Lighthouse Press.

Panic Attacks

Wilson, R. R. (2003). *Facing panic: Self-help for people with panic attacks*. Silver Spring, MD: Anxiety Disorders Association of America.

Perfectionism

Adelson, J. L., & Wilson, H. E. (2009). *Letting go of perfect: Overcoming perfectionism in kids*. Waco, TX: Prufrock Press.

Antony, M. M., & Swinson, R. P. (1998). *When perfect isn't good enough: Strategies for coping with perfectionism*. Oakland, CA: New Harbinger.

Health Anxiety

Taylor, S., & Asmundson, G. J. G. (2004). *Treating health anxiety: A cognitive-behavioral approach*. New York: Guilford Press.

Hair Pulling

Keuthen, N. J., Stein, D. J., & Christenson, G. A. (2001). *Help for hair pullers: Understanding and coping with trichotillomania.* Oakland, CA: New Harbinger.

Woods, D. W., & Miltenberger, R. G. (Eds.). (2001). *Tic disorders, trichotillomania, and other repetitive behavior disorders: Behavioral approaches to analysis and treatment.* New York: Springer.

Parenting and Discipline (School Refusal)

Bailey, B. A. (2000). *Easy to love, difficult to discipline: The 7 basic skills for turning conflict into cooperation.* New York: HarperCollins.

Baumrind, D. (1991). The influence of parenting style on adolescent competence and substance use. *Journal of Early Adolescence, 11*, 56–95.

Brooks, R., & Goldstein, S. (2002). *Raising resilient children: Fostering strength, hope, and optimism in your child.* New York: McGraw-Hill.

Dweck, C. (2006). *Mindset: The new psychology of success.* New York: Random House.

Glasser, W. (1998*). Choice theory: A new psychology of personal freedom.* New York: HarperPerennial.

Maccoby, E. E., & Martin, J. A. (1983). Socialization in the context of the family: Parent-child interaction. In P. H. Mussen (Ed.) & E. M. Hetherington (Vol. Ed.), *Handbook of child psychology: Vol. 4 Socialization, personality, and social development* (4th ed., pp. 1–101). New York: Wiley.

Phelan, T. W. (2004). *1-2-3 magic: Effective discipline for children 2–12* (3rd ed.). Glen Ellyn, IL: ParentMagic.

Sells, S. P. (2002). *Parenting your out-of-control teenager: 7 steps to reestablish authority and reclaim love.* New York: St. Martin's Griffin.

Siegel, D., & Hartzell, M. (2003). *Parenting from the inside out: How a deeper self-understanding can help you raise children who thrive.* New York: Tarcher/Penguin

Walsh, D. (2005). *Why do they act that way? A survival guide to the adolescent brain for you and your teen.* New York: Free Press.

Walsh, D. (2007). *No: Why kids—of all ages—need to hear it and ways parents can say it.* New York: Free Press.

Selective Mutism

McHolm, A. E., Cunningham, C. E., & Vanier, M. K. (2005). *Helping your child with selective mutism: Steps to overcome a fear of speaking.* Oakland, CA: New Harbinger.

Bedwetting

Bennett, H. J. (2005). *Waking up dry: A guide to help children overcome bedwetting.* Elk Grove Village, IL: American Academy of Pediatrics.

Sensory Processing Disorder

Kranowitz, C. S. (2005). *The out-of-sync child: Recognizing and coping with sensory processing disorder* (2nd ed.). New York: Perigee.

Medication

Wilens, T. (2004). *Straight talk about psychiatric medications for kids* (Rev. ed.). New York: Guilford Press.

Recommended Books for Children

Crist, J. J. (2004). *What to do when you're scared and worried: A guide for kids.* Minneapolis, MN: Free Spirit.

Golomb, R. G., & Vavrichek, S. M. (2000). *The hair pulling "habit" and you: How to solve the trichotillomania puzzle* (Rev. ed.). Silver Spring, MD: Writers Cooperative of Greater Washington.

Huebner, D. (2007). *What to do when your brain gets stuck: A kid's guide to overcoming OCD.* Washington, DC: Magination Press.

Kendall, P. C. (1992). *Coping cat workbook.* Ardmore, PA: Workbook Publishing.

March, J. S. (2006). *Talking back to OCD: The program that helps kids and teens say "no way"—and parents say "way to go."* New York: Guilford Press.

Wagner, A. P., & Jutton, P. A., (2004). *Up and down the worry hill: A children's book about obsessive-compulsive disorder and its treatment.* Rochester, NY: Lighthouse Press.

Recommended CDs

Charlesworth, E. A. (2002). *Scanning relaxation* (Audio CD). Champaign, IL: Research Press.

Lite, L. (2006). *Indigo dreams: Relaxation and stress management bedtime stories for children, improve sleep, manage stress and anxiety* (Audio CD). Marietta, GA: Lite Books.

Organizations

American Psychological Association (APA)
750 First Street, NE
Washington, DC 20002
800-374-2721
http://www.apa.org
http://www.apahelpcenter.org

The Anxiety Disorders Association of America (ADAA)
8730 Georgia Avenue, Suite 600
Silver Spring, MD 20910
240-485-1001
http://www.adaa.org

Association for Behavioral and Cognitive Therapies (ABCT)
305 7th Avenue, 16th Fl.
New York, NY 10001
212-647-1890
http://www.abct.org

The Child Anxiety Network
http://www.childanxiety.net

National Alliance on Mental Illness (NAMI)
2107 Wilson Blvd., Suite 300
Arlington, VA 22201
800-950-6264
http://www.nami.org

National Institute of Mental Health (NIMH)
Science Writing, Press, and Dissemination Branch
6001 Executive Boulevard, Room 8184, MSC 9663
Bethesda, MD 20892
866-615-6464
http://www.nimh.nih.gov

Obsessive-Compulsive Foundation (OCF)
P.O. Box 96129
Boston, MA 02196
617-978-5801
http://www.ocfoundation.org

The Trichotillomania Learning Center, Inc.
207 McPherson Street, Suite H
Santa Cruz, CA 95060
831-457-1004
http://www.trich.org

Appendix A

Overview of the Program

This page provides an overview of the program and allows you and your child to check off when each of the chapters and exercises are completed.

Chapter	Topic	☑ DONE
Chapter 1	Anxiety: What It Is and What To Do About It	
	Exercise: Fill in the Bubbles	
Chapter 2	Making Your Team and Team Goals	
	Exercise: Making Your Team and Team Goals	
Chapter 3	Relaxing Your Body	
	Exercise: Practice Relaxation	
Chapter 4	Conquer Your Worries	
	Exercise: Self-Talk Note Cards	
Chapter 5	Changing Your Thoughts	
	Exercise: Identify and Replace Thinking Errors	
Chapter 6	Changing Your Behavior: Facing Your Fears	
	Exercise: Facing Your Fears	
Chapter 7	Keep Facing Your Fears	
	Exercise: Finish Your Ladder	
Chapter 8	Lessons Learned: Celebrate Yourself	
	Exercise: Party and Certificate	

(The parent's guide has two additional chapters: Chapter 9: Motivating Your Child and Chapter 10: Special Sections)

Appendix B

Thinking Errors Quick Reference Page

- *Catastrophizing:* visualizing disaster; thinking that the worst thing is going to happen and feeling like you wouldn't be able to handle it; asking "What if . . . "
- *All-or-Nothing:* thinking in extremes, things are either perfect or a failure; there is no middle ground—it's either one extreme or another; thinking in an inflexible way
- *Filtering:* focusing on the negative parts of a situation while ignoring the positive parts; catching all the bad parts and forgetting about the good parts
- *Magnifying:* making something seem bigger and worse than it really is; turning up the volume on anything bad
- *Shoulds:* rules that you have about how things should be; using the words "should," "must," and "ought to" to show how things should be
- *Mind Reading:* thinking you know what others are thinking, particularly what they are thinking about you; usually you will think that others are thinking negatively about you
- *Overgeneralization:* taking a single incident and thinking that it will always be this way; something happens once and you think it will always happen this way
- *Personalization:* taking something personally; making it about you when it has nothing to do with you
- *Selective Attention:* paying attention to things that confirm your beliefs about something; ignoring evidence that goes against what you believe about a particular situation
- *Probability Overestimation:* overestimating the likelihood that something bad will happen

About the Author

Bonnie Zucker, Psy.D., is a licensed psychologist with an expertise in psychotherapy with children and adolescents. She received her doctoral degree in clinical psychology from Illinois School of Professional Psychology in Chicago, her master's degree in applied psychology from University of Baltimore, and her bachelor's degree in psychology from The George Washington University.

Dr. Zucker specializes in the treatment of childhood anxiety disorders. Using a cognitive-behavioral (CBT) approach, she has helped hundreds of children become anxiety-free by teaching them coping skills, methods for challenging their faulty thinking, and how to systematically face their fears. Dr. Zucker also integrates a family systems approach in order to teach parents how to most appropriately respond to their child's anxiety disorder.

Dr. Zucker is in private practice at the National Center for the Treatment of Phobias, Anxiety, & Depression in Washington, DC, and at Alvord, Baker, & Associates in Rockville, MD. She is active in training mental health professionals on the treatment of anxiety disorders.

Anxiety-Free Kids

FOR KIDS ONLY

Companion Guide

Bonnie Zucker, Psy.D.

(That means she's a psychologist!)

Contents

Welcome to *Anxiety-Free Kids* and Dr. Zucker's "For Kids Only" Companion Guide

WELCOME to Dr. Zucker's "For Kids Only" Companion Guide to the book *Anxiety-Free Kids*! My name is Dr. Bonnie Zucker and I am a type of doctor called a *psychologist*. My job is to work with kids just like you who are having a hard time with worries and fears and help them feel better. The best thing I do to help them is to teach them how to *face their fears*. I'll talk more about this later and explain what it means. Kids usually come to see me once a week, and we talk about what makes them feel scared (it's called *therapy*). During therapy, we try to come up with ways to overcome these fears. Their mom or dad also comes in at the end of the meeting to learn how to help their child deal with being afraid and worrying. We all work together as a team. This book will help you make your own team to help you face your fears.

Your parent (or someone else who cares for you a lot) got this book for you to help you deal with times when you worry or feel scared. Worrying and being scared also is called *anxiety*. When someone has anxiety or feels scared a lot, it is not his fault, and he shouldn't feel embarrassed or ashamed. But, because feeling this way is not all that fun and really can feel bad sometimes, it is a good idea to work on these feelings and make that person better. So this is what this book is all about—helping you to feel better! Feeling better also usually means feeling stronger, and other kids who learn how to deal with their anxiety say that they feel more sure of themselves. By becoming a "master" of your anxiety, you will no longer have to be afraid or worry about bad things happening.

The information in this book is the same information I talk about with kids who meet with me in my office. Maybe you already meet with a psychologist like me, or maybe you don't. Either way, you should feel very proud of yourself for starting this program—helping yourself get better is a very grown-up thing to do!

So, let's get started!

Good luck,

Dr. Bonnie Zucker

Introduction

BEFORE we get started, let me tell you a little about how this book works. Your parent (or whoever gave this book to you) is going to be reading his or her own book that goes along with your book (it's called a *companion book*). The chapters are matched up with one another so that your parent is always reading about the same thing as you. For example, in this book, Chapter 1 is all about anxiety. In your mom or dad's book, their Chapter 1 also is about anxiety.

At the end of each chapter, there are exercises for you and your parent to do together. Sometimes these will involve questions to answer together, or suggestions on what to talk about, or you may be asked to do a short activity. Whatever it is, you will work on it with your parent. Your parent's book will tell him about these exercises, as well, and your parent will read about ways he can help you complete them. The exercises are very important and often will be fun to do!

Two last things you should know. First, while I realize that many kids are raised by stepparents, grandparents, aunts and uncles, and other loving adults, I will use words like "parents," "mom," and "dad" to describe the person who is completing this program with you. If you are one of these kids, just know that when you see me talk about your parent, mom, or dad, I mean the person who gave you this book. Whoever that person is cares about you a lot and wants to help you overcome your anxiety and feel better. Second, I will use different girls' and boys' names throughout the book as examples. This is because both girls and boys have worries and anxiety.

OK, let's get started!

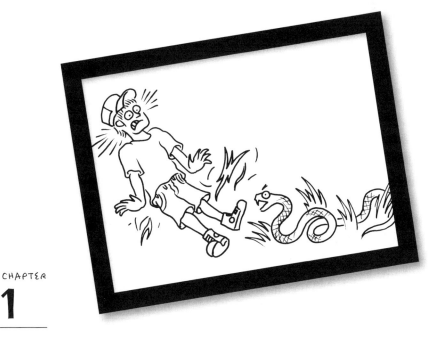

1

Anxiety

What It Is and What to Do About It

WHEN you are feeling nervous, worried, scared, or afraid, this is called *anxiety*, or feeling anxious. The opposite of feeling anxious is feeling relaxed. Everyone—kids and adults—feels nervous from time to time. Sometimes something will happen to make you feel anxious, such as when you are in a store and you cannot find your mom or dad, when you have to get a shot at the doctor's office, or when the electricity goes out and you're alone in your room. Other times, it comes out of the blue, and you just feel nervous for no reason. When this happens, you may start to worry about bad things happening. These worries usually make you feel more scared and nervous. Kids who feel scared or nervous much of the time often begin to feel bad about themselves, and worry about how well they can handle things. When you are not sure if you are able to handle something, this is called *self-doubt*. It is common to feel this way and you should not feel bad about yourself because you have anxiety and worries.

Anxiety becomes a concern when it starts to cause problems in your everyday life. For example, if your worries are preventing you from going to school, birthday parties, sleepovers, or sleeping alone at night, then it is causing a problem. If you get a lot of stomachaches or headaches, or feel like you don't have the energy to do things, it might be because of anxiety. Also, if you have trouble concentrating at school because you are focusing on your worries, then anxiety is causing a problem for you.

Let me give you some examples of kids who have anxiety:

▸ When James was 6 years old, he was in his backyard helping his father pull weeds from the garden. As he pulled out one very big weed, a garden snake jumped out at him and landed right on his stomach before it fell to the ground and glided away. Even though James was not hurt by the snake at all, after this happened, James became afraid of snakes. He began to worry about seeing another snake. Whenever he was in his backyard, he would be on guard looking for snakes. Sometimes, he would hear an animal moving in the bushes and he would run away, fearing that it was a snake in there. As he grew up, James's fear grew and grew. When he watched a scene from one of the *Harry Potter* movies that had a snake in it, he became very scared, even though the friends he was watching it with were not scared. James even refused to go to his friend's house because his friend had a pet snake. Sometimes James would feel sick to his stomach just thinking of snakes. When he turned 12, he came to therapy to learn ways to get over his fear of snakes. In therapy, he learned that he had what is called a *phobia* of snakes.

▸ Billy was a very smart 9-year-old with a great imagination. He loved to design creative games, and was always happy when he worked on his games. Even though he was one of the smartest kids in his class, Billy took a very long time to do writing assignments at school because he had a learning disability. Some of his teachers did not understand about his learning disability, and would punish him for not having all of his work done. Sometimes, his teacher even made him stay in from recess to finish his work. This made Billy feel uncomfortable and embarrassed. He started to worry about getting in trouble and having to stay back during recess. He worried so much that his muscles became all tense, he couldn't sleep at night, and he even got stomachaches and headaches. Because he felt so nervous about writing and about getting in trouble if he didn't get all of his work done, Billy would daydream and couldn't focus on his work. He worried so much that it was hard for him to concentrate. Sometimes he would be so worried that he would not want to go to school. Billy came to therapy and learned that he had what is called *generalized anxiety.*

▶ Ten-year-old Ruth spent a lot of time worrying that she would get sick. She worried that she would get sick by getting germs from others. Whenever she was at a sleepover or a party, Ruth refused to eat food from bowls that others had touched. She never ate anything homemade, especially homemade cookies or brownies, or anything from the school cafeteria. Ruth had a very hard time using public bathrooms; it was so uncomfortable for her, that she often "held it" until she got home. When she did use public bathrooms, she did her best not to touch anything there. She would flush the toilet with her foot so she didn't have to touch the flusher, and she used her sleeve to touch the faucet and door handles so she wouldn't have to touch it with her hands. If Ruth accidentally touched anything in the bathroom, even the walls of the stall, she would insist that her mother wash her clothes immediately once they got home. She wanted her mom to wash everything twice, to make sure the germs were gone. Even though she didn't really know why she was so afraid of germs, sometimes she would become so upset about getting germs on her, that she would stay at home in her room all day. Ruth's parents brought her to therapy and she learned that she had a type of anxiety called *obsessive-compulsive disorder.*

James, Billy, and Ruth all had anxiety that caused problems in their lives. All of their worries and fears were very upsetting for them, and got in the way of doing normal, everyday things, like going into the backyard, going to school, using public bathrooms, and even eating homemade cookies! Their anxiety and fears went past "normal" amounts, which they all learned was why they had to get help for their anxiety problems. All three of them got help and all three of them got over their anxiety. James, Billy, and Ruth no longer have problems with anxiety. You'll hear more about them and how they did it later in this book.

Now let me teach you the three parts of anxiety: body, thoughts, and behavior. (See Figure 1.)

Anxiety comes out in three ways: in our bodies, our thoughts, and in the way we act (our behavior). In order to understand anxiety, we need to understand the three parts of it, and we also need to learn how to make each part better. Let's go through each one.

Body

Our bodies have a reaction when we feel anxious. Different kids have different reactions, but the most common are:

- ▶ fast heartbeat;
- ▶ sweating, sweaty palms;
- ▶ difficulty breathing (shallow, fast breathing);
- ▶ tense muscles;

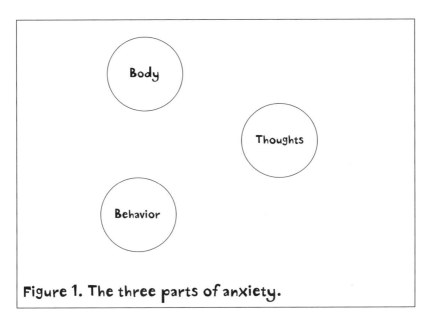

Figure 1. The three parts of anxiety.

- ▶ feeling like it's hard to swallow or you are going to choke;
- ▶ stomachaches;
- ▶ headaches;
- ▶ feeling dizzy;
- ▶ shaking; and
- ▶ feeling detached from your body.

Thoughts

When we feel anxious, we usually worry. Worry is a type of thought (for example, we think about scary things happening). Many people worry about bad things happening to them, or to someone they love. Others worry that they won't do well, like on a test, or that other kids or parents won't like them. We also might make "thinking mistakes" or "thinking errors," which are very common. These thoughts make the anxiety worse. You will learn more about thinking mistakes in Chapter 5. Also, we have negative self-talk, which involves saying things to ourselves (usually not out loud) that actually make the anxiety worse. Here are some examples of each:

- ► "What if something bad happens to my mom or dad when they go out tonight?" (worry)
- ► "What if I fail the test tomorrow?" (worry)
- ► "Other kids will laugh at me if I raise my hand and give the wrong answer." (thinking mistake)
- ► "I should get all A's in school. If I get a B, it means I am a failure." (thinking mistake)
- ► "I can't do this. I will only feel better if I go home right now." (negative self-talk)
- ► "I'm so scared, this is terrible." (negative self-talk)

Behavior

The most common behavior or action linked with anxiety and fears is avoidance. Avoidance means you don't do the thing you are afraid of or you stay away from the thing that makes you feel scared. For example, if you are afraid of dogs, you will not go near them. You may refuse to go to a friend's house if he has a dog, or you may leave a park if there are dogs around. If you are afraid when your parents leave the house, you will try to make them stay and not leave. If you are afraid of talking to other kids at school or of raising your hand and talking in front of the class, you will not do these things. Other common anxious or nervous behaviors include: reassurance-seeking (this is a fancy way of saying that you get others, usually your parents, to tell you things that make you feel better), fidgeting or being restless (for example, moving around a lot, not being able to sit still), picking or pulling (for example, your nails, your hair), crying, freezing up, and having a meltdown or tantrum.

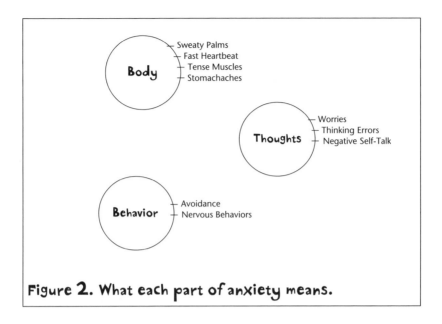

Figure **2.** What each part of anxiety means.

Now that you've learned more about the three parts of anxiety, let's look at the circles again with more detail (see Figure 2).

What to Do About Anxiety

We have to work on each part in order to best help you with your anxiety or fears. So, now that you know the three parts of anxiety, let me tell you what we're going to do with each part. For your **body**, I am going to teach you (and your parent will help, too) how to take deep, calm relaxing breaths, how to do something called *progressive muscle relaxation* (PMR for short), and how to do relaxing imagery. For your **thoughts**, you will learn positive self-talk, how to know and change your thinking mistakes, and how to conquer (or master) worry. You will learn when your thinking is realistic (likely to come true) and when it is unrealistic (not likely to come true). You also will learn how to feel better, or more confident, about yourself and your ability to handle things. For your

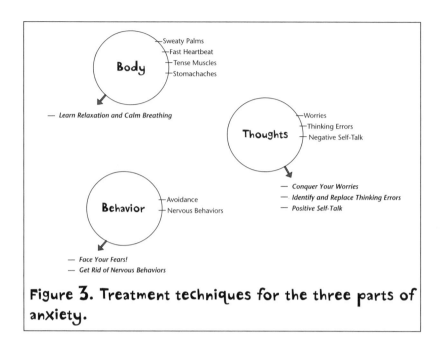

Figure 3. Treatment techniques for the three parts of anxiety.

behavior, you will learn how to face your fears so that you can overcome them and get rid of any nervous behaviors that you do.

Here are the bubbles one last time (see Figure 3).

This may sound like a lot of work, but I promise you three things:

1. It won't be nearly as hard as you think (plus we'll try to make it a little fun).
2. You will have a team to support you (I'm one of the people on your team!).
3. You definitely will feel a lot better by doing this program!

Chapter 1 Exercise
Fill in the Bubbles

Directions: You and your mom or dad will do this together. In each of the bubbles, write in the three parts of anxiety. Next to each part (bubble), write your own examples of your experience with anxiety. For example, you can write down what specific things happen to your body when you are anxious.

(*Hint:* It will end up looking a lot like the one on p. 9.)

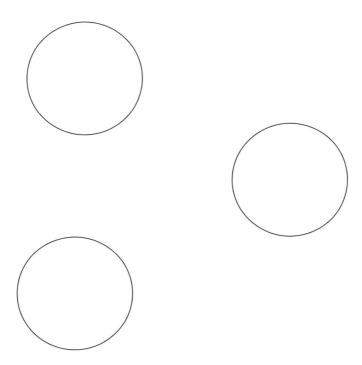

Congratulations on finishing Chapter 1! You should feel very proud of yourself because you have taken the first step in overcoming your anxiety.

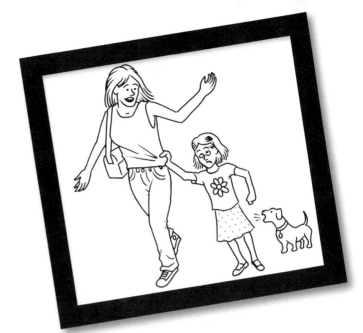

2

Making Your Team and Team Goals

THIS chapter is shorter to read than the previous one, but the exercise that you and your parent will do is longer than most of the other exercises in this book. The best part is that the exercise is going to be fun. We already talked a little about how important it is to face your fears. Let's talk more about this. As you already learned, when you avoid doing things because you are afraid or nervous to do them, this is called *avoidance behavior* because you are avoiding, or not doing, something. Each time that you don't do something because it makes you feel anxious, *the anxiety wins*. Each time you do something that makes you feel anxious, *you win and the anxiety loses*. It is you against the anxiety (You vs. Anxiety), and I promise you that as you face your fears, you *will* win!

Let me give you an example:

> Eight-year-old Thelma was one of the children I worked
> with in therapy. She was very nice, very smart, and very
> nervous about being separated from her mom. If her mom
> went out in the front of the house to take out the trash,
> Thelma would become anxious—her heart would beat fast,
> and she would stop doing whatever she was doing to go
> to the window and watch her mom. Thelma would worry
> that something bad would happen to her and that she
> wouldn't come back. Thelma also did not like to be in a
> different room than her mom, and when her mom would
> go in another room, Thelma would ask her to sing a song so
> Thelma would always know where she was. She refused to
> sleep in her own bed at night even though her mom would
> try to get her to sleep alone. Thelma would cry and cry
> and beg her mom to be able to sleep with her. Sometimes,
> Thelma's mom needed to go out without her and a babysit-
> ter would come over; this upset Thelma so much that she
> would get sick and throw up. As soon as her mom would
> come home, Thelma would feel better.

Thelma has anxiety, and her anxiety is called *separation anxiety*,
which means that she gets very nervous and worried when she is
separated from her mom, and worries about bad things happening to her mom. She does her best to *avoid* being separated from
her, because this is the thing that makes her feel so scared. Each
time that Thelma clings onto her mom and *avoids* being separated
from her, *the anxiety wins and she loses.* Even though staying near
her mom helps her to feel better at the time, it actually makes the
anxiety much worse overall. Thelma learned that she had to face
her fears to overcome them. How did she do it?

Thelma and her team (her mom, sister, and me, Dr. Zucker)
worked together to make a list of all of the things that felt scary to

her and that were hard to do. Then, Thelma and I put the list in order, from easiest to hardest, and wrote them all on a poster board, in the form of a ladder. Each step on the ladder was one of the things that was hard for her to do. Thelma learned how to relax and take deep breaths, learned that her fears were not realistic (for example, it was perfectly safe for her mom to take out the trash), and learned what to say to herself to help her deal with her scary thoughts and feelings. Thelma also learned that she was making thinking mistakes and worked on correcting them. Finally, she understood that she needed to face her fears, one step (or fear) at a time. She knew that when she was facing her fears, she would have to handle feeling some anxiety, but that the anxiety would go away with time and practice. Most importantly, Thelma was told that she would not have to take any of the steps until she was ready; Thelma would not be forced to face her fears. Instead, Thelma would be encouraged by her team to face her fear—she would be cheered on.

Thelma named her ladder "Climbing to Confidence" because she felt that her separation anxiety made her feel less confident, or sure, about herself. By facing her fears, she would feel more confident. This is what Thelma's ladder looked like:

Climbing to Confidence

(top)	Mom goes out of town without you.
	Go on a sleepover at a friend's house.
	Mom goes out for the day without you.
	Go on a play date at a friend's house.
	Mom goes out for 1 hour, then 2 hours without you.
	Mom goes out for 15 minutes, then 30 minutes without you.
	Sleep in your bed alone one night this week (then 2, 4, 5, and 7 nights).

	You use a public bathroom on your own (without mom).
	Mom takes the trash out and you stay focused on the TV.
	Mom stays upstairs while you stay downstairs (for 5, 10, 15, and 30 minutes, then for 1 hour).
	Mom goes into other rooms without singing to you.
(bottom)	You stay in living room while mom is in kitchen (for 5, 10, 15, 20, and 30 minutes).

Thelma practiced her relaxation and deep breathing, read her self-talk note cards, studied the thinking mistakes that she made and how to think more correct or realistic thoughts, and used her tools to master her worry. When she was ready, Thelma took the first step on her ladder: to go in the living room while her mom was in the nearby kitchen. She started slow, doing it for 5 minutes, then did it for longer periods of time—10, 15, 20, and 30 minutes—eventually being able to be in the living room alone for more than an hour! It was not too easy, but it wasn't nearly as hard as she thought it would be. The first time she did it, she called to her mom, who popped her head in the living room and told Thelma that she was facing her fears and doing a fantastic job. She did it again and again, and then it became very easy, and did not cause her to feel scared or nervous at all. By the third time, she did not have to ask her mom to come in, and she learned to feel comfortable being in the living room alone. She was able to relax and enjoy watching TV and reading a book. Then Thelma felt ready to take the second step: her mom would go into other rooms in the house while Thelma was in the living room or her bedroom, but her mom would not sing to her. Again, she felt nervous and scared the first time they practiced, but it got easier and easier with each practice, and soon Thelma did not feel nervous when her mom left the room. Thelma remembered to do her breathing and read her self-talk note cards. She also told herself that feeling nervous when doing the steps was normal, but that it would get better, and it did!

Like Thelma, you will learn how to face your fears. Like Thelma, you will have a ladder with your own anxieties, and will also form a team. Let's do this now!

Chapter 2 Exercise
Making Your Team and Team Goals

WHO IS ON YOUR TEAM?

Write in names of the members of your team in the blanks below. You do not have to fill in all of the blanks. Your team will be at least three people: You (the Captain), whoever is reading the parent book (usually mom or dad), and me (Dr. Zucker). Other people you can include on your team are your grandparents, sister or brother, babysitter or nanny, pets, and your therapist if you have one. Your team members all will help you to face your fears in different ways. For example, Thelma's dog, Sniffy, was on her team and Sniffy helped her face her fears by being with her in the beginning when she was nervous about her mom leaving her alone in the living room. Sniffy also gave her extra licks when she was happy about doing such a great job in facing her fears.

YOUR TEAM:

1. Team Captain: _____

                                        (your name here)

2. _____

3. _____

4. _____

5. _____

6. _____

TEAM GOALS: MAKING YOUR LADDER

You will need the following materials to make your ladder:

▶ Blank note cards
▶ Poster board (white or another light color)
▶ Markers
▶ Pen or pencil
▶ Stickers (stars, happy faces, whatever you want)

To make your ladder follow these steps:

1. Using note cards and a pen or pencil, write down all of the different things that are hard for you to do or that you avoid doing because of anxiety and worry. Your mom or dad (or both) will help you make this list. Write each of these things on a different note card. (Sometimes kids and their parents choose to write it down on a piece of paper before they write it on the note cards; either way works, just as long as each thing is written on a note card).

2. Use the floor or a table and spread out all of the note cards. Then look carefully at each of the note cards and put them in order from easiest to hardest (your parent will help). The easiest ones will be on the bottom and the hardest ones will be up at the top. Here is what Thelma's note cards looked like before she made them into a ladder:

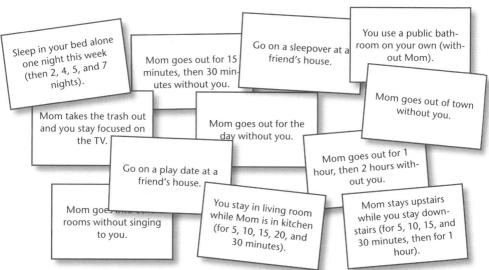

Sleep in your bed alone one night this week (then 2, 4, 5, and 7 nights).

Mom goes out for 15 minutes, then 30 minutes without you.

Go on a sleepover at a friend's house.

You use a public bathroom on your own (without Mom).

Mom takes the trash out and you stay focused on the TV.

Mom goes out for the day without you.

Mom goes out of town without you.

Go on a play date at a friend's house.

Mom goes out for 1 hour, then 2 hours without you.

Mom goes into other rooms without singing to you.

You stay in living room while Mom is in kitchen (for 5, 10, 15, 20, and 30 minutes).

Mom stays upstairs while you stay downstairs (for 5, 10, 15, and 30 minutes, then for 1 hour).

Exercises

3. Now count your note cards. How many do you have?

_____

4. Come up with a title for your ladder. Write the name here:

_____

Now write the title at the top of the poster board.

5. Use the poster board and markers to draw a great big ladder with steps underneath the place where you wrote the title. The number of steps you draw should be the same as the number of note cards you have. Leave a little space here and there in between some of the steps, just in case you decide to add more things later.

6. Write the steps, from easiest to hardest, on the ladder using the markers.

The stickers will be used once you start doing the steps. We won't begin doing this just yet; first you need to learn some tools (or ways) to deal with your anxious feelings and worries. You first will learn how to help the **body** part of anxiety. In the next chapter, you will learn about relaxation and deep breathing.

Congratulations on making your team and ladder!

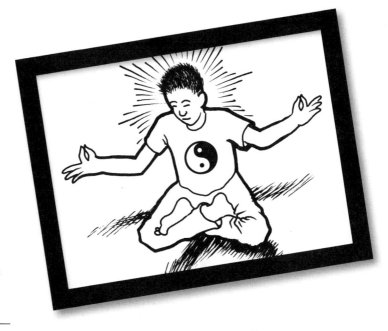

3

Relaxing the Body

I n Chapter 1, you learned that your body has a reaction when you feel anxious or afraid. In this chapter, you will learn how to relax your body and muscles (this chapter is about the body part of the three parts of anxiety). Once you practice the different types of relaxation, you will realize how good it feels to be so relaxed. With practice, you will become a master of relaxation. You also will learn that it is impossible to be relaxed and anxious at the same time. So, if you are feeling anxious and then you use your new skills to relax your body, you will not feel anxious any more.

There are three types of relaxation that we will discuss and practice:

1. calm breathing,
2. progressive muscle relaxation (PMR), and
3. relaxing imagery.

Calm Breathing

Breathing in a calm, relaxed way means that you are breathing in through your nose and out through your mouth, and the air goes all the way down to the lowest part of your belly. This is the opposite from breathing in an anxious, tense way when your breathing is shallow and the air only goes as far down as the upper part of your chest.

Try doing this: *Breathe in through your nose for 4 seconds and then out through your mouth for 4 seconds.* As you do this, try to get the air that you breathe in to go all the way to the bottom of your belly, below your belly button. It helps if you put your hands on this part of your belly and then try to get your hands to move up and down as you breathe in and out. Try not to let any air stop, or get stuck, in the top of your chest; just let the air go in easily through your nose all the way to the bottom of your belly.

Look at Thelma as she learns how to do calm breathing. Notice how her lower belly goes out as she breathes in.

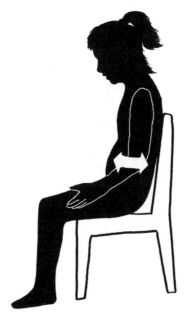

Now *breathe in through your nose for 4 seconds, hold the breath for 4 seconds, and then slowly breathe out through your mouth for 4 seconds*. It also may help to practice doing this when lying down. This way you can look at the bottom of your belly and make it rise up when you breathe in and fall down when you breathe out.

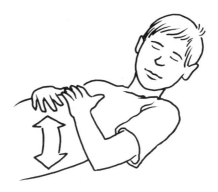

Sometimes kids will have a hard time catching their breath when they are anxious. If this happens to you, try breathing in and out through only one nostril: *Hold one of your nostrils closed and close your mouth, and breathe in and out through the one open nostril.*

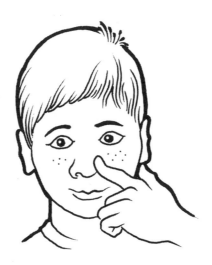

Progressive Muscle Relaxation (PMR)

PMR is a type of relaxation that involves making your muscles relax by first tightening them up and holding them for about 5–10 seconds. You do one section of your body at a time, starting with your hands and going all the way down to your feet. When you do PMR, focus on what it feels like when your muscles are tight and tense and when they are loose and relaxed. OK, let's practice:

1. Start by making tight fists, imagining that you are squeezing the juice out of a lemon. Hold your fists nice and tight and count to 10. Then let go and shake it out (shake your hands out).

2. Now pull your arms into your body, next to your ribs. Tighten up your bicep and forearms muscles, but do not make fists or tighten your hands. Hold it for 1, 2, 3, 4, 5, 6, 7, 8, 9, and 10 then let it go and shake it out. Remember to notice what your muscles feel like when they are tense and when they are loose. Sometimes after you loosen them, your muscles will feel a little tingly.

3. Bring your shoulders all the way up toward your ears and tighten them up; this should also make the back of your neck tight. Hold it for the count of 10 then allow your shoulders to drop down toward your hips. As you do this, say the word "Relax" to yourself and also breathe out slowly through your mouth.

4. Now pull your shoulders back and arch your back in toward your chest. Imagine that there is a string connected to your chest and someone is pulling the string up, lifting your chest up toward the ceiling. This will tighten your back. Hold it for a count of 10, then let it go and feel the difference between tension and relaxation.

5. Squeeze and pull your stomach, or abdominal, muscles in toward your spine. Keep it tight for 10 seconds then let it go.

6. Now squeeze your buttocks muscles (they are important, too!), and hold for 10 seconds then let go and loosen them up.

7. Stick your legs and feet straight out in front of you and point your toes in toward your chest. This will tighten the muscles in your legs and thighs. Make the muscles as tight as you can and hold for 10 seconds, then let go and allow your legs to gently drop to the ground and relax.

8. Stick your legs and feet straight out in front of you again, but this time point your toes straight out away from you and tighten up the muscles in your legs, thighs, and feet. Try to get it so you feel a little cramping in the bottom of your feet. Hold for 10 seconds then let go, allowing your legs to gently drop to the floor.

9. Now we will tighten up all of the muscles in your face. Start by clenching your teeth and jaw. Then squish up your nose, lifting it up, and close your eyes and squeeze the muscles around them, and tighten up your forehead. Hold this tightness in your whole face for 10 seconds then let go and relax. Open your mouth a little bit and move your jaw from left to right and then in circles. This will allow the jaw to become even more relaxed.

10. Last step: whole body! You want to go from being a stiff, tight robot to being a loose, relaxed rag doll. Start with tight fists, then add arms, bring shoulders up to your ears and then pull them back to tighten your back, squeeze your stomach into your spine, tighten your buttocks, put your legs out in front of you with your toes pointing out away from you and cramp up your feet, and tighten your jaw and whole face. Hold for 10 seconds (robot) and then let go (rag doll), loosening every muscle in your body. I could tell if you were a really relaxed rag doll if I tried to lift up your arm and it felt very heavy and loose.

Relaxing Imagery

Relaxing imagery is another type of relaxation, and it is best to first learn and practice it at home or in your therapist's office. You and your parent will do it together as part of the exercise at the end.

Find a comfortable place to sit or lie down. Some kids really like to use pillows, too. If you want to use pillows to get more comfortable, try putting one under your head, another one under your knees, and you also may like putting one under each of your arms. You also may enjoy listening to some relaxing music (with no words) in the background.

Once you are comfortable, I want you to *close your eyes and take a deep breath in through your nose and out through your mouth.* As you breathe in, imagine that you are breathing in clean, relaxing air and as you breathe out, let go of any stress or tension that you are holding onto. Breathing in, you let calm air go all the way down to the bottom of your belly. Breathing out, you let go of the air and your belly becomes flat. With each breath, you feel more and more relaxed. Your parent will read the following script to you, but you can also read over it to help practice getting relaxed.

Imagine that you are standing in a hallway. This is the most beautiful hallway you have ever been in—the floor is cushiony and soft, and the colors that surround you are all of your favorites. The temperature is perfect—cool but not too cool and you feel a slight breeze on your face. You notice that your body begins to loosen up.

You begin to walk down the hallway and as you do, you feel lighter and lighter. The hallway curves around to the left and then curves around to the right. As you are walking, you see that it is getting brighter and brighter, and then the hallway ends in a beautiful room.

This room is filled with windows, several of which are cracked open just a bit, allowing a nice, cool, refreshing breeze to flow through the room. Sunlight is streaming in through the windows. You walk into the room and there is a big, soft, fluffy couch up against the wall. You decide to sit and then lie down on the couch. Your body is completely supported by the couch and there is a large, fluffy pillow under your head, and another one under your knees, taking away any tension from your neck and shoulders and back and feet.

As you lie there you feel the sunlight on your body, covering you from head to toe, warming you, and you feel the cool breeze flowing over you. The combination of the warm sun and the cool breeze makes you feel even more relaxed, and you begin to fall into a deep state of relaxation. You remind yourself this is your time for relaxation. You have nowhere to go and nothing to do. Any thoughts that come into your mind simply flow in and flow out. You don't need to hold onto any thoughts—just let them flow by.

Just outside this room, there are some orange and grapefruit trees. This is a very safe, very relaxing place. Just past the trees is a beach. You begin to think about this beach, and the ocean. You imagine yourself standing at the shoreline, and can feel the wet sand as it goes in between your toes. You look out into the crystal clear water and see that there are the most beautiful fish swimming by. You look at the fish; they are all different colors—purple, turquoise, yellow, and black—and then you see a few starfish on the ocean floor. Then some beautiful stingrays swim by. You like to watch as the water changes the shape of their bodies. You are very relaxed as you watch these fish.

Then you focus on the waves, and watch as they come into the shore and then go out back into the ocean. Flowing in and then flowing out and then just flowing along. Nature is very peaceful.

Lying back on the couch, you think more about these waves. In just a moment, you will imagine a wave coming over your body, and as it does, it will soothe and comfort you, and then it will slowly leave your body, taking away any remaining tension and tightness. The wave can be any color—blue, green, purple, or it can be clear. Imagine the wave slowing going over your toes, feet, and ankles. Then it goes up your legs, knees, and thighs. It goes over your hips, hands, arms, and stomach, all the way up to your shoulders, but not over your neck. The wave is warm and comforting. It hangs out for just a minute, relaxing and soothing all of your muscles. Then the wave begins to leave, taking away all remaining tension, going down your stomach, arms, hands, and hips, all the way down past your thighs, knees, legs, and ankles, and then finally leaves your feet and toes. You are now even more relaxed.

Take a moment to enjoy this relaxation, noticing how calm and slow your breathing is. In just a minute, count to 10, and imagine yourself climbing up a set of stairs. With each step, you become more and more alert, but still very relaxed. At the top of the stairs, there will be an archway. You will walk through the archway and then you will be back in your own room, taking with you all of the feelings of relaxation.

One, take the first step.
Two, take the second step.

Three, take the third step.
Four, take the fourth step.
Five, take the fifth step.
Six, take the sixth step,
Seven, take the seventh step.
Eight, take the eighth step.
Nine, take the ninth step.
And ten, take the tenth step.

Walk through the archway, and you are back in your room. Remind yourself that you can become this relaxed anytime you'd like, and it will only take 5 minutes!

You can practice relaxing imagery with this scene or with any other relaxing scene. Your parents' book has a few more scenes like this that they'll read to you. Another thing you can do is to use your creativity and come up with your own relaxing scene! It can be anywhere you'd like—it can be a real place (maybe a place you've been) or a made-up one. The only rule is that this place needs to be free of stress and completely relaxing to you.

Stress Management

One last thing to keep in mind, because it is part of learning how to deal with anxiety, is stress management. The last part of this chapter is about how to manage or deal with stress. There are a few things that everyone should do to lower their stress beaker. What is a beaker, you ask? Well, let me explain.

A beaker is a measure of how much stress you have. Everyone always has a little bit of fluid in their beaker, the everyday kinds of things that may be annoying or stressful—like if you're having broccoli for dinner and you don't really like broccoli, or if you forget to hand in your homework, that kind of thing. Then, other things could happen that will make the level go higher. For example, you may get in trouble at home and lose the privilege of watching TV

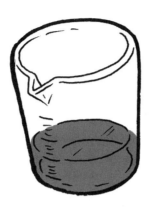

this week, or your parents have a big fight right in front of you, or you may get a bad grade on a test, or your friends were invited to a party and you weren't, or you have to get a shot and you *really* don't like shots, even more than you don't like broccoli! This is going to make the beaker level go way, way up!

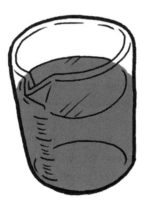

Guess what? Once your beaker is at the top, any little thing—that's right, *any little thing*—can cause it to overflow. When our beakers overflow, we explode, have a meltdown, scream, yell, and cry, whatever. And, guess what else? It's up to *you* to lower your beaker level. It's no one else's job, except yours. Even though your parents, family, and friends can help you feel better, it's really your job to make sure your beaker level doesn't go too high, and certainly doesn't overflow.

Here's what you can do to lower your beaker level:
1. Sleep well.
2. Eat well.
3. Exercise.
4. Do relaxation.
5. Express your feelings appropriately.
6. Take a hot bath, and add bubbles if you like (but not too hot).
7. Do 100 jumping jacks or push-ups (after that you'll feel too exhausted to be stressed!).
8. Write in a journal about what is bothering you and what you can do to make it better.
9. Paint a picture or do an art project.
10. Play an instrument.
11. Play with a pet (dog, cat).
12. Call a friend.
13. Distract yourself by reading a book or watching TV or a movie.
14. Ask someone to help you cook something.
15. Play outside.

You are an expert on yourself. You know what other things you can do to make yourself feel better. It is a good idea to think about some other things that make you feel relaxed, such as swinging on a swing, doing yoga, swimming or playing sports, or going outside and taking pictures with a camera. You can write some of your ideas here:

_____

_____

_____

_____

Also remember that, if you tend to worry about schoolwork and getting everything done on time, or if you have a very busy schedule, it is very important to keep up with your school demands because getting behind makes most kids feel stressed out. I also recommend that you have one day each week that you don't do ANY schoolwork, because everyone needs a break and a day to just relax and have fun. It also feels good to spend time with friends, and this can help you relax, too.

Exercises

Chapter 3 Exercise
Practice Relaxation

Your exercise this week includes:

1. A topic question for you and your mom or dad to talk about.
2. Making a calm breathing note card.
3. Practicing your relaxation 5 days this week.

Try not to think of practicing the relaxation as a chore, but as something that feels very good that you can look forward to doing. Knowing how to relax is one of the most important tools you will use when we get to the "facing your fears" part. Your mom or dad will help you by practicing with you over the week.

DISCUSSION TOPIC

Talk to you mom or dad about what makes them feel relaxed— what they do to calm down and manage stress. Tell your mom or dad what makes you feel relaxed and what you think can help you calm down. Your mom or dad might want to know what they can do to help you feel less stressed.

CALM BREATHING NOTE CARD

Use one note card to write down how to do calm breathing. Make your note card look like this one:

Calm Breathing

In → nose → 4 seconds
Hold → 4 seconds
Out → mouth → 4 seconds

Then on the back, make yours look like this:

Calm Breathing

Breathe in and out through only one nostril. Hold your other nostril closed and close your mouth.

PRACTICE RELAXATION

Check off the days that you practiced and what type of relaxation you did in the chart below.

Day of the Week	Calm Breathing	Progressive Muscle Relaxation (PMR)	Relaxing Imagery
Monday			
Tuesday			
Wednesday			
Thursday			
Friday			
Saturday			
Sunday			

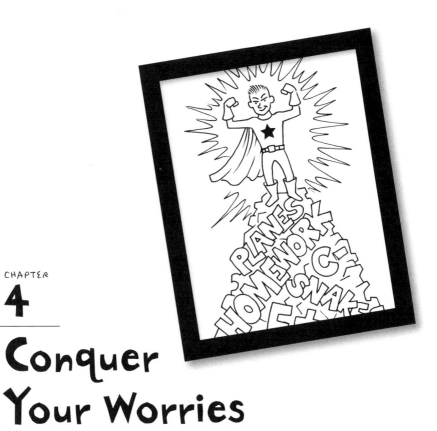

4

Conquer
Your Worries

Iɴ this chapter, you will learn how to get rid of your worries. Worries are thoughts (this chapter and the next one are about the thoughts part of anxiety). You will learn that most worrying is a waste of time.

There are six parts of conquering worry:

1. understanding the two types of worry and asking yourself two important questions,
2. getting the big picture,
3. scheduling "worry time,"
4. positive self-talk,
5. talking back to the anxiety, and
6. dealing with anticipatory anxiety.

Understanding the Two Types of Worry: Useful and Useless Worry

Useful worry is worry that helps you get something done, without causing any of the body signs of anxiety. This type of worry is productive, because it helps you produce something you want to get done. For example, when you have a big assignment in school that you really want to do well on, you spend a good amount of time working on it and worry about how good it will be. This worry is helpful because it helps motivate you to get your work done.

Useless worry is worry that prevents you from getting things done, and causes you to have body signs like tight muscles and an upset stomach. This type of worry is unproductive, because it stops you from doing something. For example, you decide not to go to a sleepover party with your friends because you are worried about being away from your mom or dad.

The most important thing that you should know about useless worry is that its goal is to make you scared and upset when there is no reason to feel this way. Useless worry is "just the anxiety talking." By facing your fears, you are going to get rid of your anxiety! You will be able to do this because when you face your fears you will see that there was nothing to worry about in the first place.

Worrying makes you feel a fake sense of control. It becomes a habit, which means you get used to thinking these worries. I know that when you look back at all of the things you have worried about, you will find that most of them never happened.

Asking Yourself Two Things

When you are worried, ask yourself the following two questions:
(1) What is the worst thing that could happen?
(2) Could I handle it?

When answering the first question, try to come up a few different possibilities. Think about what could happen and come up with a list in your head. For example, say you are worried about a test tomorrow and worried about how you will do on it. The answer to the first question might be: I would fail the test and get a lower grade in the class, and if this happened, my parents would be upset about my report card and I might get in trouble. Usually we think about what might happen and it is not really possible. For example, some kids in middle school worry that if they don't do well on one test they won't get into college, and this worry is not possible. One test will not prevent you from getting into college, plus colleges don't look at middle school report cards! Now let's say that you are worried about germs. You might think that the worst thing that could happen from touching doorknobs is that you will get germs on you, but if you thought that you would get sick and die, that would not be possible. People cannot get sick and die from touching doorknobs (if so, everyone would die because we all touch doorknobs to open doors)! So, when you think of the "worst thing that could happen," only list things that could really happen. Mom or dad or another adult can help you decide what could really happen if you are not sure.

Guess what the answer to the second question is. It starts with Y.

"Yes!" The answer is *always* "yes," because you can handle anything. There is nothing in life that you cannot handle.

Big Picture Perspective

When you are worried, try to get the "big picture" perspective by asking yourself the following:

"At the end of your very, very long and very, very wonderful life, will it really matter if _____?
Will this really matter in the big picture?" (Fill in what you are worried about.)

For example, if you are worried about a math test coming up and this worry is so strong that you can't fall asleep and are so upset that you begin to cry, try asking yourself: "At the end of my very, very long and very, very wonderful life, will it really matter if I didn't do well on this one math test in fifth grade? Will this really matter in the big picture?"

The truth of the matter is that in the big picture, it really won't matter if you didn't do well on this one test in one subject during one semester of school. Although it is important to try your best at school and study for tests, it shouldn't make you feel so upset that you are unable to sleep. Plus, you can try your best and do a great job studying for tests without feeling so upset from worries.

Let's say that you are very nervous about going to a birthday party. Maybe you are uncomfortable about going because you won't know many of the other kids there or you feel scared about separating from your mom or dad. You could ask yourself, "In the big picture of life, will it really matter if I went to this one birthday party and didn't have much fun and didn't feel very comfortable?" The truth of the matter is that in the big picture, it really won't matter if you didn't have a good time at this one birthday party. But, it is important to get yourself to go because you might have loads of fun and make new friends. More importantly, going to the party means that you are facing your fears and overcoming your anxiety. This is so important because it will help you feel better about yourself.

Schedule "Worry Time"

Another thing you can do to conquer worry is to schedule *worry time*. This means you set a time each day that you will worry on purpose. You should schedule between 15 minutes and 30 minutes for worry time, and you can do it once or twice a day. If you worry a lot, you will want to set up two times—maybe once after school and then once after dinner.

Worry time teaches you to "get your worries out" in a planned way, and you learn that you can hold off on worrying until it's time for worry time. Also, many kids figure out that their worries are the same day after day, and the worries start to seem useless and even sort of boring.

When you are doing worry time, it is very important that you use the whole time and not stop before it's over. Even if you run out of things to worry about, try to keep thinking of new things, and if you can't think of anything else, then just stay where you are until the time is up. Sometimes you will remember other worries, but sometimes you might end up just sitting there until the worry time ends.

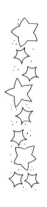

There are a few different ways to worry during worry time. You can say your worries out loud, write them down in a list, or type them up. Another thing you can do is to record yourself saying your worries (you can use a tape recorder or a digital voice recorder; your mom or dad can help with this). If you decide to record your worries, just talk into the recorder in the same way as you think when you worry. When Billy did this, he spoke into the recorder and said, "What if I can't get my work done? I'm worried that I will have to stay in for recess. What if mom doesn't let me stay home tomorrow and I have to take the test?" Billy made his worries sound just like they sounded when he thinks his worries. Once you record your worries, you can listen to the recording over and over during each worry time. Many kids end up adding onto the tape or digital recording as they think of more worries. The worry recording helps make the worries less powerful, and by listening to it over and over, you will be able to get rid of your worries!

Positive Self-Talk

Self-talk is what you say to yourself (this is part of your thoughts, so it's likely that you probably don't talk to yourself out loud). When you are feeling anxious, your thoughts are filled with worries and negative self-talk. Here are some examples of negative self-talk:

"I can't do it."
"I won't be OK."
"I need to be with mom or dad to feel safe."
"This is too scary."
"I'm too nervous to do this."

When you tell yourself these kinds of things, you will become even more nervous and scared. However, if you use positive self-talk, you will be able to get through a scary situation and you will feel less nervous and scared. Here are some examples of positive self-talk:

"I can do it."
"I can handle this."
"Everything is alright."
"I am worried, but I am OK."
"I am anxious, but I can handle it."
"I am scared, but I am safe."
"I can help myself relax."
"I must face my fears to overcome them."
"It is my choice to be calm or be nervous. I am choosing to be calm. Let me start by calming my breath."
"It is just the anxiety talking; I don't have to listen to it."

Many kids will use positive self-talk, even though they don't necessarily believe what they are telling themselves at first. But with practice, you will see that these statements are true! The more you practice this kind of self-talk, the more you will feel like you can handle situations that make you feel anxious.

Talking Back to the Anxiety

Part of self-talk is knowing how to "talk back" to the anxiety. Although it is not good behavior to talk back to your parents or teachers, or other adults, it is very good of you to talk back to the anxiety. It is important to realize that you and the anxiety are not the same. The anxiety is a separate thing, even though it often feels like it is part of you. Think of the anxiety as external or outside of you—something separate. And, when you have scary thoughts or useless worry, say to yourself, "It is just the anxiety talking" and remind yourself that you don't need to listen to it. If you listen to it, the anxiety will win and get stronger; but if you don't listen to it, you will win and get stronger!

Dealing With Anticipatory Anxiety

Anticipatory anxiety is when you feel nervous or scared about something before it happens. Anticipating something means that you are waiting for it to happen. For example, let's say that going on class field trips makes you anxious. When you hear that you are going on one tomorrow, you may be nervous and worried all day and all night, *before* the field trip occurs. In other words, you are worrying about something before it happens—and this is anticipatory anxiety. Let's say that you get very nervous when your parents go out of town, and they tell you that they are going away for the weekend. As soon as you learn about their plans, you may begin to feel very anxious and scared, even though they haven't left yet! This is called anticipatory anxiety because you are waiting for (or "anticipating") something to happen that you feel is scary.

Most of the worrying you do is about something that is *going* to happen, not something that already has happened. So, most of your worrying is really anticipatory anxiety. If you are going to see the doctor, you may worry about getting a shot. You may cry, scream, or have a meltdown, because you are so worried about the possibility of getting a shot. This is anticipatory anxiety. Once you get to the doctor's office, you may be told that you don't need any shots, or you may be told that you do need one. Let's say that you do get the shot—most kids realize that even though they don't like them, shots are not as bad as they thought they would be.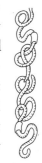

Now that you understand what anticipatory anxiety is, let me tell you what you can do to deal with it. There are three steps to dealing or coping with anticipatory anxiety:

1. Label your worries and scary feelings as anticipatory anxiety. Say to yourself, "It is just anticipatory anxiety."

2. Remind yourself that the thing you are worried about is not going to be as bad as you think it will be. The anxiety before the event is actually the worse part. For example, the field trip ends up being fun; your parents go out of town and you have a good time with whomever you stayed with (grandparents, babysitter); the shot was not fun at all, but it also wasn't the worst thing in the world and was over in a second. Also, remind yourself that the anticipatory anxiety does not make you any more prepared for dealing with the situation you are worried about. Remember, worrying makes you feel a fake sense of control. It makes you feel like you are doing something to deal with the scary situation, but really it is only making the scary situation even scarier! Anticipatory anxiety is useless worry.

3. Replace these thoughts with healthier, more balanced thoughts. Use positive self-talk to reassure yourself that you will be OK and that you can handle what comes your way!

("It might not be that bad. All of my friends will be there and I could have fun on the field trip.")

So, remember to label, remind, and replace your anticipatory anxiety.

Chapter 4 Exercise
Self-Talk Note Cards

Your exercise this week includes:
1. Making 8–10 self-talk note cards.
2. Making a list: "When the anxiety talks, it says . . ."
3. Keep practicing your relaxation (try to do it at least three times this week).

SELF-TALK NOTE CARDS

When making your note cards, you can use different colored index cards and you can add stickers to the note cards if you'd like. You can write them or have your mom or dad write them—it's your choice. You will make five note cards like the ones below, and also make three to five cards of your own (you can make more if you'd like, but try to make at least three extra cards). The ones that you make on your own should be specific to you; they should be things that you can say to yourself that will help with your own specific worries and anxieties. Your mom or dad will help you with what to write.

Here are five note cards to make (make yours look just like these)

To conquer worry, I should ask myself two things:
1. What is the worst thing that could happen?
2. Could I handle it? (answer = always yes)

It is my choice to be relaxed or do be anxious. I am choosing to be relaxed. Let me start by calming my breath.

I am scared, but I am safe.

I am uncomfortable and nervous, but I can handle it.

I don't like the anxiety, but it is not dangerous.

I must face my fears to overcome them. I am facing my fears!

I am OK.

Everything is fine.

It will all work out.

IT'S THE ANXIETY TALKING

Remember James, the boy who was afraid of snakes? Well, when his anxiety was talking, it said things like:

"Snakes are scary and they will bite you."
"Don't go near the bushes, because a snake could be in there."
"That rustling sound was a snake."
"You can't go near snakes—they are the worst!"

James had to learn how to talk back to his anxiety, and he did this by knowing when his anxiety was talking to him and choosing not to listen to it! He told himself that the anxiety was wrong; then he told himself different things to help himself be able to face his fears. For example, he told himself that the rustling sound was most likely a squirrel or a bird. He reminded himself that most snakes don't bite humans. This is how he was able to face his fears and overcome his fear of snakes.

In the space below, write in some of the things that the anxiety says when you are feeling scared or anxious:
"When my anxiety talks, it says . . ."

_____

_____

_____

_____

_____

_____

_____

_____

Exercises

RELAX

Practice your relaxation techniques three times this week. Practice with your parent and also practice alone. Try to use the calm breathing technique when you are feeling nervous or scared.

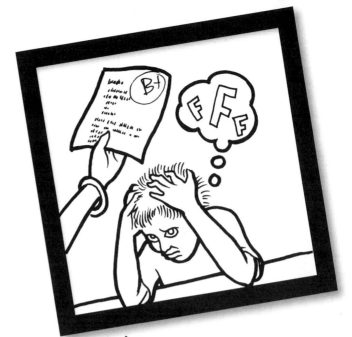

5

Changing Your Thoughts

I N this chapter, you will learn about the different types of anxious thinking. You also will learn how to change your anxious thoughts and beliefs (as a reminder, this chapter also is about the thoughts part of anxiety).

Let's start by understanding the connection between your thoughts and feelings. The way you think about a situation affects how you will feel about it. For example, if you think that playing with your neighbor's dog is a lot of fun, you will feel excited about it. But, if you think that playing with your neighbor's dog is scary and frightening, you will feel nervous about it.

Situation →	Thoughts →	Feelings
You are in front of your house and your neighbor is outside with her dog.	I really like dogs and can't wait to play with Sniffy. She's so cute!	Excited Happy Eager

Situation →	Thoughts →	Feelings
You are in front of your house and your neighbor is outside with her dog.	Dogs are so scary! I hope she doesn't come near me. If she comes toward me, I'll run inside!	Anxious Nervous Scared

Let's go through several more examples:

Situation →	Thoughts →	Feelings
You are called on in class by the teacher to answer a question.	I feel comfortable being called on. I like to share my thoughts. Maybe the teacher will like my answer.	Relaxed Calm Enthusiastic

Situation →	Thoughts →	Feelings
You are called on in class by the teacher to answer a question.	I can't stand talking in front of the class. What if I say the wrong answer and everyone laughs and thinks I'm dumb?	Anxious Nervous Scared

Situation →	Thoughts →	Feelings
You have a big science test tomorrow and you have been studying for 3 days.	I am prepared and will probably do well because I have been studying a lot.	Calm Self-Assured Organized

Situation →	Thoughts →	Feelings
You have a big science test tomorrow and you have been studying for 3 days.	What if I fail? What if I forget everything I know? I will be in big trouble if I fail. The test is going to be impossible!	Anxious Nervous Scared

The examples above show that if something makes you feel anxious, it has to do with the way you are thinking about it. This also means that you can *change the way you think to change the way you feel*! This is a very important step in overcoming your worry and anxiety. You can do this, and the more you practice, the better you will become.

Can you imagine what would happen if the child in the above example were to change his thoughts and begin thinking like a nonanxious person? So, once the thoughts about failing the science test come up (and he thinks about how hard it will be and how he will get in big trouble if he fails), he would *change* these thoughts to thoughts like "I am prepared. I will probably do well because I have been studying a lot." In the beginning, he may not believe what he is telling himself; however, as he keeps practicing this type of thinking, it eventually will become natural and automatic.

Part of changing your thoughts involves learning the type of thinking mistakes you are making that are causing you to feel anxious and nervous.

Types of Thinking Mistakes

All humans make thinking mistakes, also called thinking errors—this includes all kids and all adults. Thinking errors are thoughts that you have automatically that cause you to feel bad and anxious. Thinking errors are thoughts that are wrong or incorrect; they are rooted in anxiety. Don't feel bad for making thinking mistakes—remember, all kids and all adults make them. Let me give you a personal example:

This past year I went to an island called Barbados and heard that there were really cool sea turtles in the ocean. The only thing was that you needed to take a speed boat to get to see them. So, I arranged for the hotel's motorboat to take us to see the sea turtles. Well, when the motorboat came up to the ocean shore to pick us up, I suddenly felt a rush of anxiety and fear and worry come over me. My heart started pounding, my stomach and knees felt weak, and I couldn't stop thinking about how scary it would feel going so fast on this boat—speeding along on the ocean. I worried that I would be so scared that I'd want to come back to shore, and that I wouldn't like it at all. I really felt too afraid to go. I told my husband, Brian, that I was so nervous that I wasn't sure I could go, and asked him if he thought it would be OK. Because Brian knows that I work with kids with anxiety and that I teach kids how to face their fears, he replied, "Well, you need to face your fears," then jumped onto the boat! I decided to take his (really my) advice and got on the boat too. The next thing I knew, we were speeding along on the ocean going very fast and the funny thing was, I had no anxiety at all. Not even the tiniest amount of fear. I probably couldn't have felt afraid if I tried. I was totally calm and relaxed and loved every minute of the boat ride. I loved the feeling of the ocean air against my face, the feeling of being on a boat, traveling on water, and looking at the beautiful island as we rode by. More than all of this, swimming with the sea turtles was one of the greatest times of my life! The sea turtles were huge and so interesting to watch as they swam in their ocean. It was a magical time and it would never have happened if I didn't face my fears.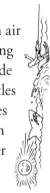

As you can see, the thoughts I had about going on the boat and my body's feelings of anxiety were not good predictors of what being on the boat would be like. My thoughts were not correct; they were wrong—they were thinking mistakes. I was making two types of thinking errors: "probability overestimations" and "catastrophizing." Sometimes one thought will actually include more than one thinking mistake.

Let me tell you about 10 different types of thinking errors and give you examples of each. Most kids tend to make several of these thinking errors. When reading about them, try to think about which ones you make:

1. **Catastrophizing:** Visualizing disaster; thinking that the worst thing is going to happen and feeling like you wouldn't be able to handle it; asking "What if . . . "
   Example: What if I am scared on the motorboat and won't be able to calm down?
   Example: You parents are going out for dinner without you and you think that something bad will happen to them or to you. What if they get hurt?

2. **All-or-Nothing:** Also known as black-and-white thinking, dichotomous thinking, and polarized thinking; thinking in extremes—things are either perfect or a failure; there is no middle ground—it's either one extreme or another; thinking in an inflexible way.

Example: If I don't get an A on this test, I will fail the whole class and have a terrible report card.

Example: You and your family planned on having pizza for dinner, but your mom brings home Chinese food instead. You are so upset and tell your mom, "The whole day is ruined now!"

3. **Filtering:** Focusing on the negative parts of a situation while ignoring the positive parts; catching all of the bad parts and forgetting about the good parts; disqualifying the positive.

Example: You go to a birthday party and have a great time until the end when another kid says something mean to you. Your dad picks you up and asks how the party was and you tell him, "It was terrible. I had the worst time!"

Example: You get your report card and make all A's and B's but got a C in history. You feel so upset and only think about your history grade; you ignore all the other good grades that you earned.

4. **Magnifying:** Making something seem bigger and worse than it really is; turning up the volume on anything bad, making it worse.

Example: Your dad reminds you that you have a check-up at the doctor's tomorrow after school. You begin to cry and you tell him that this is the worst news you have ever heard!

Example: A bug lands on your shirt and you scream at the top of your lungs and run around trying to get it off.

5. **Shoulds:** Rules that you have about how things should be; using the words "should," "must," and "ought to" to show how things should be.

Example: You make a mistake and forget to hand in an assignment. When you hand it in the next day, your teacher marks it down to a B because it is late. You feel so upset with yourself and think, "I shouldn't make mistakes like this. That was so stupid of me."

Example: A friend comes over to play and you think that she should play with whatever games you pick, because you're playing at your house. You pick out Monopoly but she tells you that she doesn't want to play Monopoly and would rather play Clue. You become very upset with her because you believe that she should follow your rules.

6. **Mind Reading:** Thinking you know what others are thinking, particularly what they are thinking about you; usually you will think that others are thinking negatively about you.

   Example: When you are answering a question in class, you think that other kids are thinking that you are stupid and don't know what you are talking about.

   Example: When your baseball coach gives you a pointer, you think that he thinks you are the worst player on the team.

7. **Overgeneralization:** Taking a single incident and thinking that it will always be this way; something happens once and you think it will always happen this way.

   Example: You give a presentation on your book report and you feel very nervous throughout the presentation. Afterward, you tell yourself that anytime you give a presentation you are going to feel very nervous.

   Example: You go to an awards ceremony at school but don't get any awards. When leaving, you tell your parents that you're never going to an awards ceremony again because you won't get an award anyway!

8. **Personalization:** Taking something personally; making it about you when it has nothing to do with you.

   Example: You walk by two girls in the lunchroom and they are whispering so you think that they are whispering about you.

   Example: You didn't receive an invitation to your friend's birthday party so you think that he must be mad at you and doesn't want to be your friend anymore.

9. **Selective Attention:** Paying attention to things that confirm your beliefs about something; ignoring evidence that goes against what you believe about a particular situation.

   Example: You think that other kids don't like you and then you remember the time you were teased at recess and when your neighbor told you she didn't want to play with you anymore. You don't think about the kids who do like you or about all of the fun you have with your friends from soccer after school.

   Example: Your brother gets a new computer and this makes you think about how your Mom and Dad don't get you anything, and how your computer is 2 years old. You don't think about how you recently got a new bed and that when you got your computer 2 years ago, your brother did not get one.

10. **Probability Overestimation:** Overestimating the likelihood that something bad will happen.

    Example: You think that your presentation is going to be terrible and that you will be panicked the whole time.

    Example: You are about to get on a motorboat and you think that you will be scared and anxious during the whole ride (does this sound familiar?).

Replacing Your Anxious Thoughts

After you have identified what your anxious thoughts are, the next step is to change them. You can do this by replacing your thoughts with balanced, neutral thoughts. For example, instead of thinking that others are thinking bad things about you, you can think that most likely they are not having bad thoughts about you. Instead of thinking about something bad happening to your parents, you can think about how they go out to dinner all of the time and are always safe. Instead of thinking that the whole day is ruined because your mom brought home Chinese food and not pizza, you can think about the day more realistically and how the rest of the day can be great (maybe not the food part, but the rest of it).

To replace your thoughts, you want to consider the facts and ask yourself, "What proof do I have that this thought is correct?" For example, what proof do you have that your mind reading is correct? How do you know that the other kids think you are stupid when you are answering a question in class? How do you know how you will feel once you are speeding along the water on a motorboat? What proof do you have that your presentation will be a disaster? Even if you have given not-so-great presentations in the past, how do you know that this particular presentation won't go well? The *fact* is that you don't have any proof about what will happen in the future, because it hasn't happened yet! Remember, your worries are part of anticipatory anxiety; they are about future events that haven't occurred yet.

Challenge your anxious thoughts by asking yourself, "What would someone who is not anxious in this situation think right now?" or "What would someone who is completely secure in this situation think right now?"

Exercises

Chapter 5 Exercise
Identify and Replace Thinking Errors

Your exercise this week includes:

1. Listing two of your anxiety situations from your ladder and the anxious thoughts you have about these situations.

2. Labeling your thinking mistakes if there are any.

3. Changing your thoughts by creating "replacement thoughts," using the tool on the next few pages to write down your old and new thoughts. Remember: Replacement thoughts are balanced and neutral thoughts that do not cause anxiety. (*Hint*: You will know that you came up with a good replacement thought when the thought makes you feel calmer and more prepared to cope with the scary situation.)

Situation →	Thoughts →	Thinking Error(s)

Replacement Thoughts:

Exercises

Situation →	Thoughts →	Thinking Error(s)

Replacement Thoughts:

Situation →	Thoughts →	Thinking Error(s)

Replacement Thoughts:

Situation →	Thoughts →	Thinking Error(s)

Replacement Thoughts:

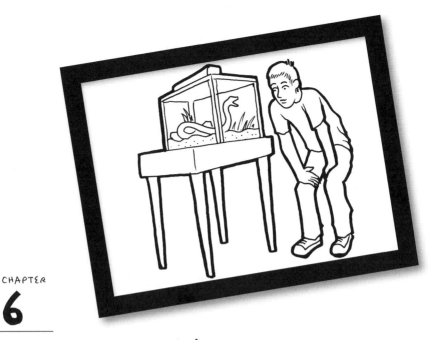

6

Changing Your Behaviors

Facing Your Fears

IN this chapter, we will focus on preparing you to face your fears! So, this chapter is about the behavior part of anxiety. You have already learned about the body and thoughts parts and are now ready for this last part: behavior.

The last chapter showed you that your thoughts impact your feelings. It also is true that your feelings impact your behavior. If you *feel* scared of something, you probably are going to try to avoid it—and avoidance is a behavior. There are other behaviors that kids often do when they are feeling scared or anxious. These include:

- ▶ reassurance seeking (asking your mom or dad or someone else to tell you that you're OK);
- ▶ clinging (staying near your parent or another adult);
- ▶ crying;

- ▸ picking (nails, hair, feet, lips, or any other part of your body);
- ▸ fidgeting (moving around a lot or playing with your fingers or hair);
- ▸ freezing up;
- ▸ having a tantrum or meltdown;
- ▸ scanning your environment (looking around for something to make you feel calmer); and
- ▸ rituals (things you do repeatedly).

As you have learned, avoiding scary situations strengthens your anxiety about the situations and your anxiety in general. To overcome your anxiety, you cannot do avoidance behavior anymore. Remember: It is you versus your fear. Take a positive attitude and tell yourself that you will win against your fears! As mentioned earlier, you will start facing your fears with the easier and less anxiety-provoking situations and then gradually move up the ladder to harder ones. When you face your fears, you are doing what is called an *exposure*, because you are exposing yourself to the scary situation.

Keep in mind that you are not going to be forced to do these exposures—you will do them as you feel ready to; however, your parent should encourage you and might give you a push to do it. Also remember that you are now better prepared to handle facing your fears. You will face your fears by using your coping tools and getting support from your parent. As you face your fears, it also is important to feel good about yourself and compliment yourself. You will reward yourself after facing each fear by putting stickers on your ladder (your parent will do this with you).

A note about getting stars/stickers on your ladder: You can earn two stars for each step on your ladder (each one goes on each side of the ladder for each step). The first star will be earned after you take the step for the first time. You will put the second star on the ladder for that step after you have practiced it enough and it doesn't make you feel anxious or scared anymore. The second star shows that you have overcome your fear for that situation.

I also have some very good news to share with you: Once you are done facing all of your fears, there will be a celebration in your honor. You and your parent(s) are going to have a little party to celebrate you and all of your hard work! You may even get an award or a special treat! You might decide to invite a sibling if you have one or a best friend or grandparent to celebrate you with you and your parent.

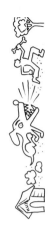

OK, so let's start facing your fears by making a **plan for coping**. A plan for coping with the exposures will help you feel prepared to do so. The exercise for this week is going to help you to remember all of the things you can do to manage or cope with your anxiety. It is normal to feel anxiety as you begin to face your fears. But, most kids find that after feeling some anxiety at first, their anxiety goes way down and usually goes away completely. It will be helpful to remind yourself of this fact. The kids I work with always feel great after facing their fears, and usually they find that it was nothing like they expected it to be—in fact, it was much easier. Finding that facing your fears isn't so bad will help motivate you to continue to face your fears that are higher on the ladder, in a step-by-step way.

Plan for Coping

A plan for coping will always include using the tools in your "toolbox." The tools are the strategies that you have learned in the previous chapters that help you deal with your anxiety. You will review the tools in your toolbox during the exercise at the end of this chapter. The tools you have include:

- ▶ calm breathing;
- ▶ progressive muscle relaxation;
- ▶ relaxing imagery;

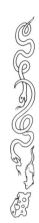

- ▸ conquer worry, including
  - ○ understanding when your worry is useless worry;
  - ○ asking yourself two things;
  - ○ finding the big picture perspective; and
  - ○ scheduling worry time;
- ▸ positive self-talk;
- ▸ talking back to the anxiety;
- ▸ dealing with anticipatory anxiety (label, remind, and replace);
- ▸ self-talk note cards (including "you must face your fears to overcome them"); and
- ▸ changing your thoughts (identifying and replacing thinking errors).

Most likely, you won't use *every* tool in your toolbox, just your favorite and most helpful ones. Plus, you may use different tools for different situations. For example, James (the boy who had a snake phobia) used calm breathing as he looked at pictures of snakes in a book but he mostly used conquer worry and positive self-talk tools when he stood near a live snake.

Sometimes kids are too nervous to use tools to conquer worry and change their thoughts. If this happens, you can use distraction techniques in addition to calm breathing to calm down enough to be able to conquer worries and change your thoughts. Examples of distraction techniques include:

- ▸ Using the ABCs to calm down: Go through the alphabet and try to come up with a different girl's name for each letter (for example, Amy, Bonnie, Camryn, Denise, Emily, Frances). Or, you could do this for boy's names, cities, countries, places, types of foods, or types of jobs (for example, artist, baker, chemist, dentist, environmentalist, firefighter). This will help distract you from the anxiety-provoking situation.

▶ Focus on something that you can see (for example, a tree, book, your sneakers) and try to think of five or more different parts of it or ways to describe it (for example, What color is it? What shape is it? What does it smell like? What does it sound like? What does it feel like? What could you use it for?).

▶ Pick a color and think of five things that come in that color.

▶ Sing a song to yourself or make up a rhyme in your head.

▶ Count backward from 100 by 7 (100, 93, 86, 79, . . .) or any other number.

Another part of making a plan for coping during exposures is to decide if you want to break down your exposure into even smaller steps. For instance, when James did his first exposure (talking about snakes) he began by talking about snakes for 1 minute, then did it again the next day for 5 minutes, then did it again on the third day for 10 minutes.

When facing your fears, review what your plan will involve. Think about which tools you will use and which distraction techniques you will rely on if you have a hard time focusing on using your tools.

When it comes time for you to do an exposure, rate how anxious or scared you were on a scale from 0 to 10. We can think of this scale as a FEAR-mometer, sort of like a thermometer that measures temperature, but this measures fear.

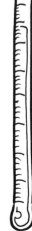

0 = no fear at all/completely relaxed like in a deep sleep

5 = nervous and scared but not too terrible

10 = extremely afraid, totally anxious, and maybe panicked

Chapter 6 Exercise
Facing Your Fears

Your exercise this week includes:

1. Drawing a picture of a toolbox and writing the different "tools" in it on your own paper (remember the tools are the different strategies you can use to manage your anxiety; they are all listed earlier in this chapter).

2. Taking the first step of your ladder (do your first exposure).
   - ► Remember to put stickers on your ladder after you have practiced your first step several times.
   - ► Remember to note what your anxiety level was on the FEAR-mometer.

Make your picture of the toolbox look something like this one:

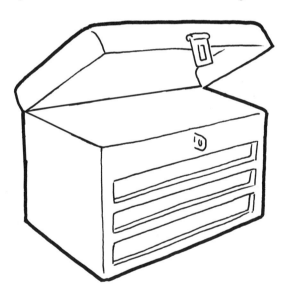

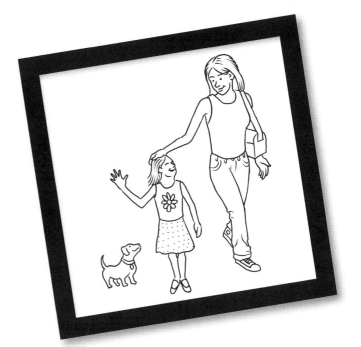

Keep Facing
Your Fears

THIS is another short chapter that also is on behavior. If you are reading this chapter, it most likely means that you have faced your first fear, so let me say "Congratulations!" This was a big step and you should feel very proud of yourself for getting this far. I am certainly proud of you!

As you can probably guess, the exercise at the end of this chapter is going to be taking the rest of the steps on your ladder, one at a time. Once you finish taking all of the steps on your ladder, you can go onto the next chapter (which is the last chapter) and celebrate.

Remember that although it is going to be hard to do many of the steps on your ladder, you will feel so much better once you do them and you will be free to live your life without anxiety controlling it. You also will feel better about yourself. Before we talk more about the behavior part, let's talk a little about the idea of feeling proud of yourself.

Self-esteem refers to how you feel about yourself and it can either be good (healthy) or bad (unhealthy). Kids with good self-esteem feel proud of themselves and their accomplishments and they know what they are good at doing. Also, they don't forget how good they are when things don't work out well for them. For example, they don't beat themselves up for their mistakes or when they don't do as well as they would like to do. And, when others say mean things about them, like some kids do, they don't believe it—they don't forget that they are a good, special person. Like anxiety, which has three parts, self-esteem also has three parts:

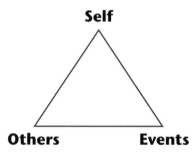

- ▶ The "Self" part, which is the most important of the three parts, means that you know and own your strengths; you know what is wonderful and special about you and you remember these qualities even on bad days. You know what you are good at doing, whether it's playing an instrument, dancing, or being a great athlete or an excellent speller.

- ▶ The "Others" part means that other people can help you feel good about yourself; your parents, friends, and teachers can compliment you or show they care about you and this will make you feel good about yourself. They can support you and help you know your positive strengths and areas to work on and improve upon. For example, your teacher can help you understand what your strengths are and also ways to become even better at your schoolwork.

▶ The "Events" part means that certain things can happen to you or certain things that you do can help you feel great about yourself; facing your fears counts as one of these events. Other examples are when you study hard for a test and earn an A or when you score a goal for your team, or when you earn a green belt in karate.

When facing your fears, it is very important to cheer yourself on and encourage yourself to do the thing you are afraid of. It is very important to know your success as you go along and how you are mastering your worries by facing your fears. Remember that the anxiety tries to get you to doubt yourself (make you feel unsure about yourself), and when you face your fears you are proving it wrong! Tell yourself that you can do it and that you will succeed. Remind yourself that others believe in you—they know that you can do it, too. I *know* that you can do it and I *know* that once you face your fears, you will win the battle against your anxiety!

When facing your fears, try to stay mostly in the order of your ladder. Sometimes you will skip around, but it's usually not a good idea to do the steps at the top until you've done some of the ones at the bottom or the middle. Most kids find that it's best to do the steps close to their order on the ladder, although sometimes they will do a step a little ahead. This is perfectly fine, as long as you feel ready for it. For example, you may get the chance to do one of your steps, like getting invited to a party (if going to a party is on your ladder), and you might want to take advantage of the chance to do it. Again, this is OK as long as you feel like you are mostly ready to do it. Feeling ready doesn't mean that you will feel no anxiety about doing it; it just means that you are willing to try, and maybe you can picture yourself doing it. Also, most kids find that it gets much easier to face their fears as they go through the steps.

This also is a good time to work on your nervous behaviors that you read about in Chapter 6. Examples of nervous behaviors include asking your mom or dad to tell you a situation will work out alright (called reassurance-seeking), clinging, and checking things like if the dog is safe or if the doors are locked. The goal is to get rid of these behaviors. I know it can be very hard to stop doing these behaviors because you are used to doing them, but getting rid of them is part of overcoming your worry and anxiety.

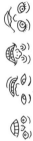

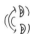

Your mom or dad will help you stop doing the nervous behaviors by reminding you when you are doing them and by not answering questions when you are seeking reassurance from them. Mom and dad are not doing this to upset you or as a punishment. Your parents' book explains that your mom and dad need to stop telling you that everything will be OK because it makes the anxiety and worry stronger. When your mom or dad tells you that it will be OK (gives you reassurance), it makes you feel better right now, but makes your anxiety and worry worse in the long-term. Instead, your parent will ask you to use your self-talk and relaxation tools to help yourself feel better.

Also, you and your mom or dad may decide to use a calendar to track each day that you don't use your nervous behaviors. For example, at night, Billy would repeatedly ask his mom if he could stay home from school the next day; sometimes she would let him. After coming to therapy, Billy's mom learned that letting him stay home from school was actually making his anxiety worse. His mom then learned to change the way she responded to Billy, and instead she would say to Billy, "You sound nervous about going to school, but you have to go. What can you do to calm down, and how can I make it better for you?" At first, Billy didn't like this response from his mom, but after a while he got used to it. They used a calendar and every night that Billy didn't ask his mom if he could stay home from school, she would give him a check or a put a sticker on his calendar. He began to see that everything would be fine, even though his mom didn't let him stay home from school. Billy realized that he felt better about himself when he was able to handle his anxiety and worries on his own.

Like Billy, you can get rid of your nervous behaviors and feel better about yourself. Take a minute to think about what nervous behavior you do most often, and tell yourself that you will work on getting rid of it. Getting rid of your nervous behaviors is one of the last parts of overcoming anxiety.

When you take the rest of the steps of your ladder, come up with more replacement thoughts to help you change the way you think about each situation. Try to figure out which thinking mistake you may be making, and then come up with a new, more balanced thought. Remember that you can change the way you think to change the way you feel. The exercise at the end includes a chart that you can use to come up with replacement thoughts for the different steps. Also, don't forget to use the tools in your toolbox; you can look back at the picture of your toolbox in Chapter 6 for a review.

One last note about taking the rest of the steps on your ladder: When kids take a step on their ladder, they don't just do it once and then forget about it. Instead, they continue to do it over and over until it no longer makes them feel anxious or scared. This also is important for you to do. So, once you do something on your ladder, you should continue to do it repeatedly. It soon will become something that you are able and comfortable to do! When you take the rest of the steps on your ladder, you may feel anxious and scared when you do them at first, but I promise that as you continue to practice, it will get easier and easier. Plus, many kids find that they aren't anxious or scared at all when they take one of their steps, and they realize that it was just their anticipatory anxiety talking.

Good luck with taking the rest of your steps!

Chapter 7 Exercise
Finish Your Ladder

Take the next step on your ladder, and then the next step, and so on, until you've taken them all. Remember to go at your own pace, but try to do 1–2 steps each week.

Don't forget to:

▶ put stickers on your ladder next to the step after you've taken it, and

▶ note what your anxiety level was on the FEAR-mometer.

Change the way you think to change the way you feel! Use steps from your ladder for the chart below (write them under "situation") and write down the automatic thought or worry you have about facing that fear. Then, figure out which thinking error you might have used, and come up with a new, more balanced and accurate thought for your replacement thought. Your parents can help you come up with these new thoughts. When you take each step, try to remind yourself of the replacement thought you came up with for that situation. Good luck!

Exercises

Situation →	Thoughts →	Thinking Error(s)

Replacement Thoughts:

Exercises

Situation →	Thoughts →	Thinking Error(s)

Replacement Thoughts:

Situation →	Thoughts →	Thinking Error(s)

Replacement Thoughts:

Situation →	Thoughts →	Thinking Error(s)

Replacement Thoughts:

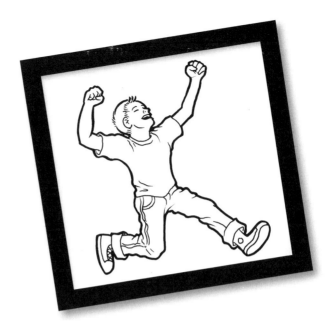

8

Lessons Learned

Celebrate Yourself

WELCOME to the last chapter of this book! Getting to this chapter is a *great* thing to have done and you deserve a big cheer: "Hurray! Great job! You did it!" You have faced your fears and *won!* In other words: Congratulations!

You deserve a party (and you're going to have one very soon) to celebrate all of your hard work and for trying your very best and overcoming your fears. Now, before you have a celebration with your family, there are two very last things to talk about:

1. What lessons did you learn?
2. How can you handle anxiety and worries if they come up again in the future?

Lessons Learned

So, how did you do it? Let's review what you did to get to the point of facing your fears and overcoming your anxiety.

First, you learned about the three parts of anxiety: body, thoughts, and behavior. After creating your team and team goals and making your ladder, you learned how to work on each of the three parts to overcome your anxiety. To help your body's feelings of anxiety, you learned and practiced:

1. calm breathing,
2. progressive muscle relaxation, and
3. relaxing imagery.

To help with your anxious thoughts, you learned:

1. how to master your worries;
2. how to use positive self-talk;
3. about the situation-thought-feeling connection (how you think will affect how you feel, so changing your thoughts can change the way you feel); and
4. about thinking errors and how to change them into healthy replacement thoughts.

Finally, to help with the behaviors part, you learned how to face your fears, one by one, and you did it. You also learned how to get rid of nervous behaviors and worked on those too. Changing the way you think not only changed the way you feel, but it also changed the way you behaved.

By facing your fears, you learned that you can win and overcome your anxiety and take charge of it. Kids who face their fears also often learn that their fears were not as bad as they expected them to be. Once they were in the different situations, they found out it wasn't that bad after all. They learned that they can face their fears.

You also learned that when something difficult or challenging comes your way, you can face it and become stronger as a result. Most kids who face their fears also realize that they feel better about themselves and then their self-esteem improves and becomes stronger. You learned that you can believe in yourself and your abilities to face your fears.

Handling Worry and Anxiety in the Future

Most kids who complete this program and face their fears don't go back to being as anxious and nervous as they were in the beginning. Now that you have read this book and done the exercises, you hopefully are not feeling anxious like you did when you started. But, it is always a good idea to know what to do in case you get a little anxious from time to time, or get really anxious about something different. Well, the best part is: you *know* what to do, because you just did it as you read this book. You can handle any anxiety in the future in the same way that you handled your anxiety during this program. So, even if things come up for you, you can use all of these skills to deal with it, and not allow it to become a problem. You are now an expert on how to handle any anxiety in the future.

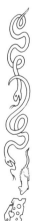

Let me give you an example: James successfully overcame his fear of snakes by completing this program. More than a year went by without thinking about or worrying about snakes when James went to a birthday party and there was a snake trainer there to put on a show (can you believe it?). Because he had not thought about snakes for so long, when he first saw the huge snake around the neck of the trainer, James suddenly felt a rush of fear. For a moment, he forgot that he was no longer scared of snakes! Then he realized that he knew what to do: He knew that he needed to stay at the party, and actually sat closer to the snake trainer to make it more like he was facing his fears. He also took a few deep breaths and remembered that he could handle this. He reminded himself that he would be OK and that he's done this before so he can do it now. After about 5 minutes, James felt back to normal again. He was calm and felt no fear. James was reminded that whenever he felt anxious, he just needed to use the tools in his toolbox and face his fears.

Like James, you may have some anxiety and worry from time to time. Just do what you have throughout this program, and you'll be fine. Keep this book someplace safe and come back to it whenever you need to. I know that it will all work out for you, and wish you all the best in your future.

Congratulations again and good luck!

Chapter 8 Exercise
Celebrate Yourself With a Party
and Earn Your Official Certificate of Achievement

Talk to your mom or dad about the party and who should come to it. Some kids have the party with just their parents, and others invite their siblings, pets, or friends. There is no right or wrong way to do it—the only rule is that you have fun and celebrate all of your hard work and success!

For the Certificate of Achievement, your parent will fill in the information and you can decorate it anyway you like. Have a great party—you deserve it!

Exercises

Certificate of Achievement

We Hereby Certify That

_____

Has Overcome

_____

Granted On _____

Authorized by _____

Appendix A

Overview of the Program

This page provides an overview of the program and allows you and your parent to check off when each of the chapters and exercises are completed.

Chapter	Topic	☑ DONE
Chapter 1	Anxiety: What It Is and What To Do About It	
	Exercise: Fill in the Bubbles	
Chapter 2	Making Your Team and Team Goals	
	Exercise: Making Your Team and Team Goals	
Chapter 3	Relaxing Your Body	
	Exercise: Practice Relaxation	
Chapter 4	Conquer Your Worries	
	Exercise: Self-Talk Note Cards	
Chapter 5	Changing Your Thoughts	
	Exercise: Identify and Replace Thinking Errors	
Chapter 6	Changing Your Behavior: Facing Your Fears	
	Exercise: Facing Your Fears	
Chapter 7	Keep Facing Your Fears	
	Exercise: Finish Your Ladder	
Chapter 8	Lessons Learned: Celebrate Yourself	
	Exercise: Party and Certificate	

Appendix B

Thinking Errors Quick Reference Page

- *Catastrophizing:* visualizing disaster; thinking that the worst thing is going to happen and feeling like you wouldn't be able to handle it; asking "What if . . . "
- *All-or-Nothing:* thinking in extremes, things are either perfect or a failure; there is no middle ground—it's either one extreme or another; thinking in an inflexible way
- *Filtering:* focusing on the negative parts of a situation while ignoring the positive parts; catching all the bad parts and forgetting about the good parts
- *Magnifying:* making something seem bigger and worse than it really is; turning up the volume on anything bad
- *Shoulds:* rules that you have about how things should be; using the words "should," "must," and "ought to" to show how things should be
- *Mind Reading:* thinking you know what others are thinking, particularly what they are thinking about you; usually you will think that others are thinking negatively about you
- *Overgeneralization:* taking a single incident and thinking that it will always be this way; something happens once and you think it will always happen this way
- *Personalization:* taking something personally; making it about you when it has nothing to do with you
- *Selective Attention:* paying attention to things that confirm your beliefs about something; ignoring evidence that goes against what you believe about a particular situation
- *Probability Overestimation:* overestimating the likelihood that something bad will happen